SUPPLEMENTS DESK REFERENCE
by Jen O'Sullivan

Supplements

DESK REFERENCE

JEN O'SULLIVAN

❦

I am forever grateful to my team of researchers and editors: Caite Bellavia, Cindy Edens, Danah Meyers, Mary White, Michelle Hancock, Stephanie Ward, and Tara Adams. Without their help this book would have never been published. I am blessed to know you all and love doing life with you. A special extra thanks to Caite Bellavia who helped keep us all in line and who is the queen of fact checking, and to Tara Adams who kept me in line with content and formatting. You are all a blessing to me!

To my husband, who loves me even when my brain checks out as I am writing, and to my son, who always tells me he loves me as he walks by my office. My two men give me the energy to keep moving forward and Jesus is the reason for everything! Without Jesus, literally I would be lost. Thank you for being my guide, my teacher, my corrector, my warrior, my friend, and the lover of my soul. Thank you, Holy Spirit, for your guidance and words, and thank you, Father, for blessing me with breath and life upon life.

❧

OVERVIEW

The "Supplements Desk Reference" by Jen O'Sullivan, covers all 52 of Young Living's® supplements. It contains specific protocols using Young Living's® recommended directions for support areas such as hormones, liver support, bone health, glucose, cholesterol, gluten allergies, weight management, stress, and sleep, along with the basics of child, dog, cat, and horse health. The SDR contains a comprehensive list of common allergens along with a complete list of all the vitamins, minerals, enzymes, amino acids, and herbs found in the Young Living® products and which supplements that contain them. When you need to know what the best supplement is to take, in order to get more vitamin D, you will be able to know the answer right away... it's OmegaGize3™.

DISCLAIMER

This is very important and you will see this statement several times throughout this book.
The protocols and supplement descriptions in this book are based off of the usage descriptions from the Young Living® website and information readily available online. The amount and timing of each dosage are based off of the label on each product. In some instances, lower doses are recommended in this book. When you start a new supplement regimen, it is important to start slowly and pay close attention to your body. Everyone's body is unique and will respond differently. If a product does not work for you, please try another one. Check with your doctor if you are taking prescription medications. Pharmaceutical drugs should not be consumed at the same time as natural supplements. It is best to give a four hour buffer between them. Always consult your doctor when you start a new regimen.

This book gives suggestions on how to support healthy systems. It is not intended to treat or diagnose existing conditions or illnesses. Each supplement consists of multiple ingredients. Each ingredient that is listed has a basic description of what it is commonly used for in the medical and holistic practice industries. Herbs and roots have been used for centuries and the traditionally studied uses for each are readily found on sources such as PubMed, Science Direct, the National Center for Biotechnology Information, U. S. National Library of Medicine, and the Food and Drug Administration websites.

The content in this book has not been evaluated by the FDA and the supplements and protocols will not treat or cure any sickness or disease. The author is not a doctor and has published this book as a means to have a compilation of information, in one spot, to make it easier to understand the many supplements Young Living® carries.

CONTENTS

CJ

Thank you, Gary Young, for creating these gems!

Gary Young first added essential oils to the supplements MultiGreens™ and ComforTone® in 1984. Gary was a pioneer. He pushed the natural supplement market forward with great force, yet with incredible ease because he was armed with his powerful essential oils. Young Living® is the only company on the planet to carry a full line of herbal and whole-food based nutrition infused with true botanical essential oils.

"Here's to the crazy ones, the misfits, the rebels, the troublemakers, the round pegs in the square holes…the ones who see things differently—they're not fond of rules…You can quote them, disagree with them, glorify, or vilify them, but the only thing you can't do is ignore them because they change things…they push the human race forward, and while some may see them as the crazy ones, we see genius, because the ones who are crazy enough to think that they can change the world are the ones who do." - Steve Jobs

SO

INTRODUCTION

We live in a world where supplementation is the norm. We take vitamin C in mass doses, get vitamin B injections, and if you're not on a full-spectrum multivitamin, your mother might just cut you out of her will, if she finds out. Dietary supplements were not a major thing until the U.S. Congress passed the Dietary Supplement and Health Education Act (DSHEA) of 1994.[1] After that, dietary supplement consumption skyrocketed. In the United States alone, the supplement market is a $31 billion dollar industry. Seventy-six percent of all adults in the United States take some form of dietary supplement, as of 2017.[2] It is estimated that there are 80 to 90 thousand dietary supplement products on the market, as of 2016, according to PBS producer, Priyanka Boghani.[3]

The scary reality from the FDA, regarding all of these supplements, can be understood by the following quotes from the FDA.[4]

- "Federal law does not require dietary supplements to be proven safe to FDA's satisfaction before they are marketed."
- "For most claims made in the labeling of dietary supplements, the law does not require the manufacturer or seller to prove to the FDA's satisfaction that the claim is accurate or truthful before it appears on the product."
- "Dietary supplement manufacturers do not have to get the agency's [FDA's] approval before producing or selling these products."

Supplements are exactly what the word means: to add an extra amount of what we are not getting in our nutrition. Whole food nutrition is the most important aspect to proper health, and the goal is to get as much of that nutrition as possible from what God has created. The reality is, the food sources we currently have access to are very different from those that our grandparents, or even our parents, grew up consuming.

We have massively depleted our soils, but more importantly, even if you are able to get organic, farmer's market type produce and proteins, they are usually picked far before they should be, or the animals are fed from sources that are not ideal. Did you know most produce is picked about two weeks before it is ripe? Did you also know that often the most vital phyto-nutrients (plant nutrients) are developed during the last few days of ripening?

It is unfortunate, but the reality is, we do not get the right vitamins, minerals, micro minerals, and nutrients in the everyday food sources we eat. Supplementation is a great way to go, but sadly most supplements are synthetic or so isolated that your body does not know what to do with them, so you end up having the supplements you paid good money for go in one end and out the other, without even getting into your system to be used. The act of something going into your body and your body using it is called "bioavailability."

Around 90% of the supplements you can buy today are not fully bioavailable, because they are synthetic.[5] When you consume a synthetic, your body does not know what to do with it. You will simply urinate and defecate your money right down the toilet. Young Living® is different for a couple of reasons. First, they use whole food sources in fruits, veggies, herbs, and roots for their supplements. Second, they infuse many of their supplements with essential oils. Essential oils are extremely volatile and very small in their molecular structure, making them an excellent vehicle, or pathway, to increase the bioavailability of the supplements.

The essential oils themselves are different than any you can purchase on the market because they are the whole distillation, allowing for a true "entourage effect," which basically means that because the essential oil has not been modified, and the whole of the oil is used, there is much greater action, or synergy, that occurs within the oil, and therefore, within our bodies. Most companies practice what is called "fractional distillation" with their essential oils, simply because the final product smells better and is easier to market to the masses.

With these two important factors in place — whole plant nutrition infused with unaltered essential oils — you will get dietary supplementation through Young Living® that is second to none. Young Living® offers three types of nutritional supplements: Foundation, Cleansing, and Targeted.

Foundation Nutrition
Noted by the green labeled bottles, the Foundation Nutrition products are the vitamins and minerals that support a healthy lifestyle.

Cleansing Nutrition
Noted by the blue labeled bottles, the Cleansing Nutrition products are specifically designed to support the detox and cleansing of the body.

Targeted Nutrition

Noted by the orange labeled bottles, these are formulated with specific ingredients including powerful Essential Oils to support specific nutritional needs. These supplements target everything from enzyme support and joint health, heart, brain, and hormone support.

The following is a list of all the supplements, in alphabetical order, that Young Living® carries to date, as more are added each year. All essential oil ingredients are 100% pure, therapeutic-grade essential oil from Young Living®.

SOURCES

1. https://www.ncbi.nlm.nih.gov/books/NBK216048/
2. https://www.crnusa.org/resources/2017-crn-consumer-survey-dietary-supplements
3. https://www.pbs.org/wgbh/frontline/article/can-regulators-keep-up-with-the-supplements-industry/
4. https://www.fda.gov/consumers/consumer-updates/fda-101-dietary-supplements
5. https://myersdetox.com/90-of-vitamins-are-synthetic/

THE SUPPLEMENTS

- Vitality™ Essential Oils
- AgilEase™
- AlkaLime®
- Allerzyme™
- AminoWise™
- BLM™
- Balance Complete™
- CardioGize™
- ComforTone®
- CortiStop®
- Detoxzyme®
- Digest & Cleanse™
- EndoGize™
- Essentialzyme™
- Essentialzymes-4™
- FemiGen™
- ICP™
- ImmuPro™

- Inner Defense™
- JuvaPower®
- JuvaTone®
- K & B™
- KidScents MightyPro™
- KidScents MightyVites™
- KidScents MightyZyme™
- Life 9™
- Longevity Softgels™
- Master Formula™
- MegaCal™
- MindWise™
- Mineral Essence™
- MultiGreens™
- NingXia NITRO®
- NingXia Red®
- NingXia Zyng™
- OmegaGize3™

- PD 80/20™
- ParaFree™
- PowerGize™
- Prostate Health™
- Pure Protein™ Complete
- Rehemogen™
- SleepEssence™
- Slique® Bars
- Slique® CitriSlim
- Slique® Essence Oil
- Slique® Shake
- Sulfurzyme®
- Super B™
- Super C™ (Chewable)
- Super C™ (Tablet)
- Super Cal™ Plus
- Thyromin™

DISCLAIMER

The protocols and supplement descriptions in this book are based off of the usage descriptions from the Young Living® website and information readily available online. The amount and timing of each dosage are based off of the label on each product. In some instances, lower doses are recommended in this book. When you start a new supplement regimen, it is important to start slowly and pay close attention to your body. Everyone's body is unique and will respond differently. If a product does not work for you, please try another one. Check with your doctor if you are taking prescription medications. Pharmaceutical drugs should not be consumed at the same time as natural supplements. It is best to give a four hour buffer between them. Always consult your doctor when you start a new regimen.

This book gives suggestions on how to support healthy systems. It is not intended to treat or diagnose existing conditions or illnesses. Each supplement consists of multiple ingredients. Each ingredient that is listed has a basic description of what it is commonly used for in the medical and holistic practice industries. Herbs and roots have been used for centuries and the traditionally studied uses for each are readily found on sources such as PubMed, Science Direct, the National Center for Biotechnology Information, U. S. National Library of Medicine, and the Food and Drug Administration websites.

The content in this book has not been evaluated by the FDA and the supplements and protocols will not treat or cure any sickness or disease. The author is not a doctor and has published this book as a means to have a compilation of information, in one spot, to make it easier to understand the many supplements Young Living® carries.

SECTION ONE

the protocols

- Essential Oil Protocols Using Vitality™ Oils
- General Health Protocol
- Aging Gracefully Protocol
- Bone Health Protocol
- Brain Health and Cognition Protocol
- Cholesterol Support Protocol
- Colon Cleanse Protocol
- Digestive, Gut, and Colon Health Protocol
- Energy Support Protocol
- Emotional Support Protocol
- Glucose Support Protocol
- Gluten Support Protocol
- Healthy Hair, Skin, and Nails Protocol
- Hormone Health General (Women) Protocol
- Hormone Health General (Men) Protocol
- Hormone Health (Women) - Menopause & Fertility Support Protocol
- Hormone Health - Adrenal Support Protocol
- Hormone Health - Thyroid Support Protocol
- Immunity Protocol
- Joint and Mobility Health Protocol
- Liver Support Protocol
- Stress & Sleep Support Protocol
- Urinary Support Protocol
- Weight Support Protocol
- Kid's Health Protocol - General Health
- Kid's Health Protocol - Immunity Support
- Dog Health Protocol - Healthy Coat
- Dog Health Protocol - Mobility Support
- Dog Health Protocol - Digestive Support
- Cat Health Protocol
- Horse Health Supplements

ESSENTIAL OIL PROTOCOLS USING VITALITY™ OILS

The Vitality™ line of essential oils through Young Living® are designed specifically for consumption. They are labeled as dietary supplements, in accordance with the FDA labeling regulations and guidelines. These oils are considered GRAS which means Generally Recognized (or Regarded) as Safe for consumption, which are known essential oils used in food additives and flavorings as well as for therapeutic use. When consumed, essential oils support our body systems. The following body systems are supported by the internal use of essential oils labeled for consumption through the Young Living® Vitality™ line.

- Circulatory
- Digestive and Gut
- Endocrine
- Immunity
- Integumentary
- Lymphatic
- Nervous
- Renal/Urinary
- Respiratory

You may use the Vitality™ line in capsules (preferred method), in liquids such as water or juice, as rectal (suppository), or vaginal (pessary) inserts. You may even add these oils to your food. To get the full therapeutic value from them, it is recommended that you use them in capsule form. There are two main types of capsules to consider: regular veggie capsules that dissolve in your stomach that you can buy directly from Young Living® or at a health food store, or a longer dissolving veggie capsule that dissolves in your stomach and intestines. The longer dissolving ones are harder to find. A good source is through AromaReady.com called "Design Release" capsules. Size 00 is larger and will carry around 14 drops of liquid. Size 0 is smaller and will carry around 10 drops.

There are two types of Vitality™ line essential oil capsules you may make: daily capsules and bomb capsules. Daily capsules may be created using around 3-5 drops of essential oil for daily support. Bomb capsules may be created using around 8-10 drops to create a "bomb" for your system. A "bomb" is a stronger capsule intended to give you more aggressive support. Bombs should only be used 1-2 times over the course of 4-8 hours and only once per month. Please do not use bombs to treat sickness or disease, and always consult your doctor if you are sick. Daily capsules and bombs are meant to help support your terrain, meaning they strengthen your already healthy systems, protecting them from dipping below the wellness line. Lastly, do not take multiple capsules for multiple systems at the same time. Give at least 4 hours between capsules and do not take more than 2 per day.

The following pages give some examples of typical daily capsules along with detailed instructions explaining how to make them and store them. You should not take multiple recipes at the same time. Pay close attention to how your body responds. You may rotate these recipes or create your own. See page 72 for more details and the Vitality Usage Guide on page 198. Always be your own best advocate for your health and consult your doctor if you choose to make any major adjustments in your health care regime.

CIRCULATORY SYSTEM CAPSULES

Circulatory System Daily Capsule Recipes using Vitality™
GENERAL CIRCULATORY
- Recipe: 2 drops Cinnamon Bark, 1 drop Peppermint, 1 drop Lemon
- Recipe: 2 drops Orange, 1 drop Black Pepper, 1 drop Lemongrass
- Recipe: 1 drop Clove, 1 drop Rosemary, 1 drop Tangerine
- Recipe: 2 drops Marjoram, 1 drop Dill, 1 drop Fennel, 1 drop Oregano
- Recipe: 2 drops Lemongrass, 1 drop Tarragon, 1 drop Lavender
- Recipe: 2 drops Lavender, 1 drop Nutmeg, 1 drop Thyme

HEART HEALTH
- Recipe: 2 drops Orange, 1 drop Oregano, 1 drop Thyme

BLOOD HEALTH
- Recipe: 2 drops Tarragon, 1 drop Rosemary, 1 drop Orange
- Recipe: 2 drops Ocotea, 1 drop Marjoram, 1 drop Lemon
- Recipe: 1 drop Lemongrass, 1 drop Fennel, 1 drop Clove

Directions
Using a 0 or 00 size veggie capsule, add the desired recipe, then top off with a minimum of 4 drops olive or grapeseed carrier oil. Consume with 4-8 oz of water.

Storage
You may create multiple capsules ahead of time or create one each day. Keep in the freezer in a labeled glass container.

How long should you use these capsules?
- Do not take multiple recipes at the same time. Use only one for a couple days and then rotate through a few to see what works best for your body.
- There are two types of Vitality™ line essential oil capsules you may make: daily capsules and bomb capsules.
- Daily capsules may be created as the recipe states and used for daily support.
- Bomb capsules may be created using double or triple the recipes to create a "bomb" for your system. A "bomb" is a stronger capsule intended to give more aggressive support. Bombs should only be used 1-2 times over the course of 4-8 hours and only once per month. Please consult your doctor if you are sick.
- Daily capsules and bombs are meant to help support your terrain, meaning they strengthen your already healthy systems, protecting them from dipping below the wellness line.
- Do not take multiple capsules for multiple systems at the same time. Give at least 4 hours between capsules.

DIGESTIVE SYSTEM CAPSULES

Digestive System Daily Capsule Recipes using Vitality™

GENERAL DIGESTION
- Recipe: 3 drops DiGize™
- Recipe: 3 drops JuvaFlex™
- Recipe: 3 drops JuvaCleanse™

LIVER
- Liver Recipe: 2 drops Dill, 1 drop Cardamom, 1 drop Sage, 1 drop Coriander
- Liver Recipe: 3 drops JuvaCleanse™, 1 drop Rosemary
- Liver Recipe: 3 drops GLF™, 1 drop Carrot Seed
- Liver Recipe: 2 drops Rosemary, 1 drop Tangerine, 1 drop Celery Seed

GALLBLADDER
- Gallbladder Recipe: 2 drops Lemon, 1 drop Spearmint, 1 drop Oregano
- Gallbladder Recipe: 2 drops Lime, 1 drop Peppermint, 1 drop Jade Lemon™
- Gallbladder Recipe: 2 drops German Chamomile, 1 drop Lime

COLON
- Colon Recipe: 2 drops Thyme, 1 drop Fennel, 1 drop Cardamom
- Colon Recipe: 2 drops Tarragon, 1 drop Cinnamon Bark, 1 drop Peppermint

PANCREAS
- Pancreas Recipe: 2 drops Coriander, 1 drop Cinnamon Bark
- Pancreas Recipe: 1 drop Coriander, 1 drop Lemon, 1 drop Peppermint

Directions
Using a 0 or 00 size veggie capsule, add the desired recipe, then top off with a minimum of 4 drops olive or grapeseed carrier oil. Consume with 4-8 oz of water.

Storage
You may create multiple capsules ahead of time or create one each day. Keep in the freezer in a labeled glass container.

How long should you use these capsules?
- Do not take multiple recipes at the same time. Use only one for a couple days and then rotate through a few to see what works best for your body.
- There are two types of Vitality™ line essential oil capsules you may make: daily capsules and bomb capsules.
- Daily capsules may be created as the recipe states and used for daily support.
- Bomb capsules may be created using double or triple the recipes to create a "bomb" for your system. A "bomb" is a stronger capsule intended to give more aggressive support. Bombs should only be used 1-2 times over the course of 4-8 hours and only once per month. Please consult your doctor if you are sick.
- Daily capsules and bombs are meant to help support your terrain, meaning they strengthen your already healthy systems, protecting them from dipping below the wellness line.
- Do not take multiple capsules for multiple systems at the same time. Give at least 4 hours between capsules.

ENDOCRINE SYSTEM CAPSULES

Endocrine System Daily Capsule Recipes using Vitality™
HORMONE HEALTH
- Recipe: 3 drops SclarEssence™
- Recipe: 2 drops Bergamot, 1 drop Nutmeg
- Recipe: 3 drops Lavender, 1 drop Sage, 1 drop Fennel

ENERGY SUPPORT
- Recipe: 2 drops Grapefruit, 1 drop Black Pepper, 1 drop Ginger
- Recipe: 2 drops Lemon, 1 drop Nutmeg, 1 drop Mountain Savory
- Recipe: 1 drop Lemongrass, 1 drop Jade Lemon™, 1 drop Peppermint

METABOLISM SUPPORT
- Recipe: 1 drop Grapefruit, 1 drop Cinnamon Bark
- Recipe: 1 drop Spearmint, 1 drop Lime, 1 drop Black Pepper

SLEEP & FOCUS SUPPORT
- Recipe: 2 drops Lavender, 1 drop Lime
- Recipe: 2 drops Frankincense, 2 drops Copaiba, 1 drop Tangerine

Directions
Using a 0 or 00 size veggie capsule, add the desired recipe, then top off with a minimum of 4 drops olive or grapeseed carrier oil. Consume with 4-8 oz of water.

Storage
You may create multiple capsules ahead of time or create one each day.
Keep in the freezer in a labeled glass container.

How long should you use these capsules?
- Do not take multiple recipes at the same time. Use only one for a couple days and then rotate through a few to see what works best for your body.
- There are two types of Vitality™ line essential oil capsules you may make: daily capsules and bomb capsules.
- Daily capsules may be created as the recipe states and used for daily support.
- Bomb capsules may be created using double or triple the recipes to create a "bomb" for your system. A "bomb" is a stronger capsule intended to give more aggressive support. Bombs should only be used 1-2 times over the course of 4-8 hours and only once per month. Please consult your doctor if you are sick.
- Daily capsules and bombs are meant to help support your terrain, meaning they strengthen your already healthy systems, protecting them from dipping below the wellness line.
- Do not take multiple capsules for multiple systems at the same time. Give at least 4 hours between capsules.

These statements have not been evaluated by the Food and Drug Administration.
Young Living® products are not intended to diagnose, treat, cure, or prevent any disease.

IMMUNE SYSTEM CAPSULES

Immune System Daily Capsule Recipes using Vitality™
- Recipe: 3 drops Thieves®, 1 drop Oregano
- Recipe: 3 drops Frankincense, 1 drop Orange, 1 drop Lavender
- Recipe: 2 drops Lemongrass, 2 drops Copaiba, 1 drop Basil
- Recipe: 1 drop Cinnamon Bark, 1 drop Clove, 1 drop Bergamot
- Recipe: 2 drops Lavender, 1 drop Frankincense, 1 drop Oregano
- Recipe: 2 drops Bergamot, 1 drop Basil, 1 drop Thyme, 1 drop Lemon
- Recipe: 1 drop Rosemary, 1 drop Peppermint, 1 drop Black Pepper
- Recipe: 2 drops Clove, 1 drop Lemon, 1 drop Lavender

Directions
Using a 0 or 00 size veggie capsule, add the desired recipe, then top off with a minimum of 4 drops olive or grapeseed carrier oil. Consume with 4-8 oz of water.

Storage
You may create multiple capsules ahead of time or create one each day. Keep in the freezer in a labeled glass container.

How long should you use these capsules?
- Do not take multiple recipes at the same time. Use only one for a couple days and then rotate through a few to see what works best for your body.
- There are two types of Vitality™ line essential oil capsules you may make: daily capsules and bomb capsules.
- Daily capsules may be created as the recipe states and used for daily support.
- Bomb capsules may be created using double or triple the recipes to create a "bomb" for your system. A "bomb" is a stronger capsule intended to give more aggressive support. Bombs should only be used 1-2 times over the course of 4-8 hours and only once per month. Please consult your doctor if you are sick.
- Daily capsules and bombs are meant to help support your terrain, meaning they strengthen your already healthy systems, protecting them from dipping below the wellness line.
- Do not take multiple capsules for multiple systems at the same time. Give at least 4 hours between capsules.

These statements have not been evaluated by the Food and Drug Administration.
Young Living® products are not intended to diagnose, treat, cure, or prevent any disease.

INTEGUMENTARY SYSTEM CAPSULES

Integumentary System Daily Capsule Recipes using Vitality™
SKIN
- Recipe: 2 drops Carrot Seed, 1 drop Frankincense, 1 drop Lavender
- Recipe: 3 drops Orange, 1 drop German Chamomile, 1 drop Coriander
- Recipe: 2 drops Copaiba, 2 drops Clove

HAIR
- Recipe: 1 drop Frankincense, 1 drop Orange, 1 drop Peppermint
- Recipe: 2 drops Rosemary, 1 drop Lavender

NAILS
- Recipe: 2 drops Lemon, 1 drop Lavender, 1 drop Frankincense
- Recipe: 1 drop Copaiba, 1 drop Jade Lemon™, 1 drop Lavender

Directions
Using a 0 or 00 size veggie capsule, add the desired recipe, then top off with a minimum of 4 drops olive or grapeseed carrier oil. Consume with 4-8 oz of water.

Storage
You may create multiple capsules ahead of time or create one each day. Keep in the freezer in a labeled glass container.

How long should you use these capsules?
- Do not take multiple recipes at the same time. Use only one for a couple days and then rotate through a few to see what works best for your body.
- There are two types of Vitality™ line essential oil capsules you may make: daily capsules and bomb capsules.
- Daily capsules may be created as the recipe states and used for daily support.
- Bomb capsules may be created using double or triple the recipes to create a "bomb" for your system. A "bomb" is a stronger capsule intended to give more aggressive support. Bombs should only be used 1-2 times over the course of 4-8 hours and only once per month. Please consult your doctor if you are sick.
- Daily capsules and bombs are meant to help support your terrain, meaning they strengthen your already healthy systems, protecting them from dipping below the wellness line.
- Do not take multiple capsules for multiple systems at the same time. Give at least 4 hours between capsules.

LYMPHATIC SYSTEM CAPSULES

Lymphatic System Daily Capsule Recipes using Vitality™
- Recipe: 1 drop Thieves®, 1 drop Grapefruit
- Recipe: 2 drops Lemongrass, 1 drop Lime, 1 drop Lemon
- Recipe: 1 drop Nutmeg, 1 drop Lime
- Recipe: 1 drop Rosemary, 1 drop Grapefruit
- Recipe: 2 drops Peppermint, 1 drop Lemon, 1 drop Nutmeg

Directions
Using a 0 or 00 size veggie capsule, add the desired recipe, then top off with a minimum of 4 drops olive or grapeseed carrier oil. Consume with 4-8 oz of water.

Storage
You may create multiple capsules ahead of time or create one each day. Keep in the freezer in a labeled glass container.

How long should you use these capsules?
- Do not take multiple recipes at the same time. Use only one for a couple days and then rotate through a few to see what works best for your body.
- There are two types of Vitality™ line essential oil capsules you may make: daily capsules and bomb capsules.
- Daily capsules may be created as the recipe states and used for daily support.
- Bomb capsules may be created using double or triple the recipes to create a "bomb" for your system. A "bomb" is a stronger capsule intended to give more aggressive support. Bombs should only be used 1-2 times over the course of 4-8 hours and only once per month. Please consult your doctor if you are sick.
- Daily capsules and bombs are meant to help support your terrain, meaning they strengthen your already healthy systems, protecting them from dipping below the wellness line.
- Do not take multiple capsules for multiple systems at the same time. Give at least 4 hours between capsules.

These statements have not been evaluated by the Food and Drug Administration.
Young Living® products are not intended to diagnose, treat, cure, or prevent any disease.

NERVOUS SYSTEM CAPSULES

Nervous System Daily Capsule Recipes using Vitality™
GENERAL NERVOUS SYSTEM
- Recipe: 3 drops Orange, 1 drop Frankincense, 1 drop Lavender
- Recipe: 2 drops Lavender, 1 drop Peppermint

BRAIN
- Recipe: 1 drop Peppermint, 1 drop Thyme, 1 drop Cardamom
- Recipe: 2 drops Orange, 1 drop Lemongrass, 1 drop Lavender
- Recipe: 2 drops Frankincense, 2 drops Thyme

Directions
Using a 0 or 00 size veggie capsule, add the desired recipe, then top off with a minimum of 4 drops olive or grapeseed carrier oil. Consume with 4-8 oz of water.

Storage
You may create multiple capsules ahead of time or create one each day. Keep in the freezer in a labeled glass container.

How long should you use these capsules?
- Do not take multiple recipes at the same time. Use only one for a couple days and then rotate through a few to see what works best for your body.
- There are two types of Vitality™ line essential oil capsules you may make: daily capsules and bomb capsules.
- Daily capsules may be created as the recipe states and used for daily support.
- Bomb capsules may be created using double or triple the recipes to create a "bomb" for your system. A "bomb" is a stronger capsule intended to give more aggressive support. Bombs should only be used 1-2 times over the course of 4-8 hours and only once per month. Please consult your doctor if you are sick.
- Daily capsules and bombs are meant to help support your terrain, meaning they strengthen your already healthy systems, protecting them from dipping below the wellness line.
- Do not take multiple capsules for multiple systems at the same time. Give at least 4 hours between capsules.

These statements have not been evaluated by the Food and Drug Administration.
Young Living® products are not intended to diagnose, treat, cure, or prevent any disease.

RENAL SYSTEM CAPSULES

Renal System Daily Capsule Recipes using Vitality™
RENAL SYSTEM GENERAL
- Recipe: 2 drops Carrot Seed, 2 drops Lemon, 1 drop Lavender
- Recipe: 1 drop Fennel, 1 drop Citrus Fresh™
KIDNEY
- Recipe: 2 drops Grapefruit, 1 drop Orange, 1 drop Copaiba
- Recipe: 2 drops Copaiba, 1 drop Jade Lemon™, 1 drop Tangerine
BLADDER
- Recipe: 1 drop Thyme, 1 drop Lime, 1 drop Copaiba, 1 drop Orange
- Recipe: 1 drop Clove, 1 drop Lemon, 1 drop Rosemary
- Recipe: 2 drops Mountain Savory, 1 drop Lemongrass, 1 drop Lavender
URINARY TRACT
- Recipe: 2 drops Celery Seed, 1 drop Tarragon, 1 drop Lemon
- Recipe: 2 drops Fennel, 1 drop Copaiba, 1 drop Lavender

Directions
Using a 0 or 00 size veggie capsule, add the desired recipe, then top off with a minimum of 4 drops olive or grapeseed carrier oil. Consume with 4-8 oz of water.

Storage
You may create multiple capsules ahead of time or create one each day. Keep in the freezer in a labeled glass container.

How long should you use these capsules?
- Do not take multiple recipes at the same time. Use only one for a couple days and then rotate through a few to see what works best for your body.
- There are two types of Vitality™ line essential oil capsules you may make: daily capsules and bomb capsules.
- Daily capsules may be created as the recipe states and used for daily support.
- Bomb capsules may be created using double or triple the recipes to create a "bomb" for your system. A "bomb" is a stronger capsule intended to give more aggressive support. Bombs should only be used 1-2 times over the course of 4-8 hours and only once per month. Please consult your doctor if you are sick.
- Daily capsules and bombs are meant to help support your terrain, meaning they strengthen your already healthy systems, protecting them from dipping below the wellness line.
- Do not take multiple capsules for multiple systems at the same time. Give at least 4 hours between capsules.

These statements have not been evaluated by the Food and Drug Administration.
Young Living® products are not intended to diagnose, treat, cure, or prevent any disease.

RESPIRATORY SYSTEM CAPSULES

Respiratory System Daily Capsule Recipes using Vitality™
- Recipe: 2 drops Peppermint, 2 drops Frankincense, 1 drop Lavender
- Recipe: 2 drops Lavender, 2 drops Lemon, 2 drops Peppermint
- Recipe: 2 drops Thieves®, 1 drop Ginger, 1 drop Copaiba, 1 drop Peppermint
- Recipe: 2 drops Copaiba, 1 drop Laurus Nobilis, 1 drop Lemongrass
- Recipe: 2 drops Lemongrass, 1 drop Oregano, 1 drop Rosemary, 1 drop Lime
- Recipe: 2 drops Cardamom, 1 drop Lavender, 1 drop Peppermint

Directions
Using a 0 or 00 size veggie capsule, add the desired recipe, then top off with a minimum of 4 drops olive or grapeseed carrier oil. Consume with 4-8 oz of water.

Storage
You may create multiple capsules ahead of time or create one each day. Keep in the freezer in a labeled glass container.

How long should you use these capsules?
- Do not take multiple recipes at the same time. Use only one for a couple days and then rotate through a few to see what works best for your body.
- There are two types of Vitality™ line essential oil capsules you may make: daily capsules and bomb capsules.
- Daily capsules may be created as the recipe states and used for daily support.
- Bomb capsules may be created using double or triple the recipes to create a "bomb" for your system. A "bomb" is a stronger capsule intended to give more aggressive support. Bombs should only be used 1-2 times over the course of 4-8 hours and only once per month. Please consult your doctor if you are sick.
- Daily capsules and bombs are meant to help support your terrain, meaning they strengthen your already healthy systems, protecting them from dipping below the wellness line.
- Do not take multiple capsules for multiple systems at the same time. Give at least 4 hours between capsules.

These statements have not been evaluated by the Food and Drug Administration.
Young Living® products are not intended to diagnose, treat, cure, or prevent any disease.

GENERAL HEALTH PROTOCOL

The General Health Protocol is a basic, healthy lifestyle protocol that everyone 12 years and older can benefit from. It covers all your bases for optimal dietary supplementation. You may add targeted nutrition items such as Sulfurzyme™, a hormone support like FemiGen™, or any other Young Living® supplement that is right for you.

Supplements for this Protocol
- NingXia Red®
- Master Formula™
- MultiGreens™
- Life 9™
- OmegaGize3™
- Essentialzymes-4™
- Super Cal™ Plus (optional for additional plant derived calcium)
- Super B™ (optional for additional B support)

IDEAL SUPPLEMENT SCHEDULE

Breakfast
- NingXia Red® - drink 1-2 ounces with breakfast.
- Master Formula™ - Take all 4 capsules with breakfast.
- OmegaGize3™ - Take 2 capsules with breakfast.
- Super B™ - Take one tablet with breakfast.
- Super Cal™ Plus - Take 2 capsules with breakfast.

Lunch
- Essentialzymes-4™ - Take 2 capsules (one dual dose blister pack) just before lunch.
- Super B™ - Take 1 tablet with lunch.
- MultiGreens™ - Take 3 capsules with lunch.

Dinner
- Essentialzymes-4™ - Take 2 capsules (one dual dose blister pack) just before dinner.
- MultiGreens™ - Take 3 capsules with dinner.
- OmegaGize3™ - Take 2 capsules with dinner.

After Dinner
- Life 9™ - Take 1 capsule 2-3 hours after dinner on an empty stomach. Do not take with any internal essential oils.

How long should you use this protocol?
Every person's needs are different and everyone's situation is different. Some may need to take this type of protocol every day for the rest of their lives, while others may only need it during certain seasons. Please be your own best advocate and always check with your doctor before starting or stopping any specific regimen.

These statements have not been evaluated by the Food and Drug Administration. Young Living® products are not intended to diagnose, treat, cure, or prevent any disease.

AGING GRACEFULLY PROTOCOL

As we age our bodies start to decline. There are several things you can do to keep your systems working well. It is encouraged to also continue to move by getting 15-20 minutes of walking per day and eating lots of fruits and veggies. Below is a simple protocol that you are welcome to add onto, such as a probiotic like Life 9™ or a hormone supporting supplement such as PD 80/20™. If you are currently taking prescription drugs, make sure you check with your doctor before starting this protocol. It is recommended that you do not take these natural supplements with your prescriptions. Give a minimum of 4 hours between natural supplements and prescribed drugs.

Supplements for this Protocol
- NingXia Red®
- Longevity Softgels™
- Master Formula™
- Super Cal™ Plus
- OmegaGize3™
- AgilEase™
- Sulfurzyme™ capsules or powder

IDEAL SUPPLEMENT SCHEDULE

Breakfast
- NingXia Red® - drink 1-2 ounces with breakfast.
- Master Formula™ - Take all 4 capsules with breakfast.
- OmegaGize3™ - Take 2 capsules with breakfast.
- Super Cal™ Plus - Take 2 capsules with breakfast.

Between Breakfast and Dinner
- AgilEase™ - Take 2 capsules.
- Sulfurzyme™ - Take 2-3 capsules or 1/2 teaspoon powder with juice or water.

Dinner
- Essentialzymes-4™ - Take 2 capsules (one dual dose blister pack) just before dinner.
- Longevity Softgels™ - Take 1 capsule with dinner.
- OmegaGize3™ - Take 2 capsules with dinner.

How long should you use this protocol?
Every person's needs are different and everyone's situation is different. Some may need to take this type of protocol every day for the rest of their lives, while others may only need it during certain seasons. Please be your own best advocate and always check with your doctor before starting or stopping any specific regimen.

These statements have not been evaluated by the Food and Drug Administration.
Young Living® products are not intended to diagnose, treat, cure, or prevent any disease.

BONE HEALTH PROTOCOL

As we age, bone density becomes more and more important to consider. There are multiple types of calcium and the key is to know what they are used for as well as how much calcium is actually in the supplement. The amount in each supplement is called Elemental Calcium. It can be a little confusing to figure out what is what in the world of calcium, but the key is to choose one based on your personal needs. Young Living® has products that contain calcium ascorbate, calcium carbonate, dicalcium phosphate, calcium fructoborate, and calcium citrate. The most common calcium supplements are Calcium Carbonate and Calcium Citrate.

- Calcium Carbonate is what is taken to help ease stomach acid. You find this in antacids to help with heartburn and stomach acid. It contains about 40% of elemental calcium. It is known to cause constipation.
- Calcium Citrate is what is used when stomach acid is low. It is a gentler form of calcium and is easier to absorb.
- Calcium Fructoborate is a natural derivative of boron. Boron is an important mineral to support bone density and reduce inflammation.
- Dicalcium Phosphate is not a technical source of calcium but is used by doctors and herbalists to help repair joints.
- Calcium Ascorbate is essentially vitamin C with about 10% calcium. People use this as it is a gentler form of calcium and will not cause gas. It is easily absorbed and you do not need to eat food with it. The downside is the small amount of calcium per serving.

While supplementation is often necessary, the best form of calcium is getting it from your diet. The most bioavailable forms are from non-animal sources such as seeds (poppy, sesame, and chia), beans, lentils, almonds, spinach, kale, seaweed, and figs. While these foods have a low RDI (recommended daily intake) of calcium, these sources are far more bioavailable than isolated supplements such as calcium carbonate and calcium citrate.

There is another form of calcium that is not often found in supplements but is something that outshines all supplements you can find. Super Cal™ Plus from Young Living® contains a synergistic blend of bioavailable calcium, magnesium, and trace minerals. These are derived from red algae that is harvested off the coast of Iceland. When you truly want to support your bones, you need to make sure you have calcium, magnesium, D3, and K2. Super Cal™ Plus has it all. To support even more, consider bumping up your mineral intake and also get some extra D3.

There are some lifestyle choices that can cause loss of calcium. Two factors that cause excess calcium elimination are caffeine and sodium. Limit these when using this protocol. Also, be sure to not take these natural supplements at the same time as pharmaceuticals. Give a 4 hour buffer before or after.

Supplements for this Protocol
- Super Cal™ Plus (for calcium, magnesium, D3, and K2)
- Mineral Essence™ (for magnesium and boron)
- OmegaGize3™ (for D3)

IDEAL SUPPLEMENT SCHEDULE

Breakfast
- Super Cal™ Plus - Take 2 capsules with breakfast.
- OmegaGize3™ - Take 2 capsules with breakfast.
- Note: do not take Mineral Essence™ with Super Cal™ Plus as it may compromise the absorption of zinc and iron found in Mineral Essence™.

Lunch
- Optional: Mineral Essence™ - Add 5 half-droppers (1ml each) as a shot or in 5 capsules with dinner.

Dinner
- OmegaGize3™ - Take 2 capsules with dinner.
- Mineral Essence™ - Add 5 half-droppers (1ml each) as a shot or in 5 capsules with dinner.

How long should you use this protocol?
Every person's needs are different and everyone's situation is different. Some may need to take this type of protocol every day for the rest of their lives, while others may only need it during certain seasons. Please be your own best advocate and always check with your doctor before starting or stopping any specific regimen.

These statements have not been evaluated by the Food and Drug Administration.
Young Living® products are not intended to diagnose, treat, cure, or prevent any disease.

NOTES:

BRAIN HEALTH & COGNITION PROTOCOL

The brain is a massively complex organ that should not be overlooked when considering your overall health. Consider how profound the brain is. Our memory, thought process, ability to move and think, sight, speech, emotions, and logic all rely on the brain. Loss of any one of these functions would be catastrophic for most of us, yet we often take them for granted until they are gone.

Consider supporting your brain naturally by eating a diet rich in omega-3s, such as salmon and tuna, antioxidant-rich berries like blueberries and strawberries, broccoli, nuts, avocados, and other healthy items rich in antioxidants and healthy fats. Also, make sure to get at least 15-30 minutes of exercise at least five times a week. The added benefits to your brain when you simply take a walk every day are exceptionally powerful.

There are also some things to stay away from, such as processed sugar, alcohol, processed foods, and interestingly, staying up late and not getting enough sleep. Out of all of these, getting enough sleep is the most important thing to help support your brain. Most people need 7-9 hours of sleep per night, and the average American gets 6.8 hours of sleep. Over time, this will compound upon itself causing sleep deprivation. Sleep deprivation causes memory loss and a slower functionality rate in motor skills. It is important to consider these tips when working on improving your brain health.

The Brain Health & Cognition Protocol features products known to help support cardiovascular and cognitive health. The ingredients in this protocol support memory function, focus, and overall brain health.

NOTES:

Supplements for this Protocol
- MindWise™ Sachets
- OmegaGize3™
- Super B™
- CardioGize™
- NingXia Red®
- NingXia NITRO™

IDEAL SUPPLEMENT SCHEDULE

Breakfast
- CardoGize™ - Take 2 capsules before breakfast.
- NingXia Red® - Drink 1-2 ounces with breakfast.
- OmegaGize3™ - Take 2 capsules with breakfast.
- Super B™ - Take 1 tablet with breakfast.
- MindWise™ß Sachets - Take 1 sachet just after breakfast.

Lunch
- NingXia Red® - Drink 1-2 ounces with lunch.
- NingXia NITRO® - Drink 1 tube with lunch. (optional as needed)
- Super B™ - Take 1 tablet with lunch.
- OmegaGize3™ - Take 2 capsules with lunch.

Note: Do not take CardioGize™ if you are on blood thinning medication.

How long should you use this protocol?
Every person's needs are different and everyone's situation is different. Some may need to take this type of protocol every day for the rest of their lives, while others may only need it during certain seasons. Please be your own best advocate and always check with your doctor before starting or stopping any specific regimen.

These statements have not been evaluated by the Food and Drug Administration.
Young Living® products are not intended to diagnose, treat, cure, or prevent any disease.

NOTES:

CHOLESTEROL SUPPORT PROTOCOL

Cholesterol is a waxy particle found in the blood. There is good and bad cholesterol. The liver creates 75% of cholesterol we have in our body, while 25% comes from food sources. Cholesterol is necessary for healthy cells and to help the cells do their job correctly.

Good cholesterol (HDL) is responsible for taking cholesterol from the cells to the liver. The liver will then break down the cholesterol and pass it out of the body in the feces. Bad cholesterol (LDL) takes cholesterol from the liver back into the cells. While cholesterol in the cells is necessary, a build up can cause health issues such as a restriction of blood and oxygen to the organs.

The liver cleans toxins from our body and eliminates them through urine from the kidneys. In the case of cholesterol, the liver eliminates it through the colon. Supporting the liver and the digestive process through a diet high in fiber-rich veggies, good fats, such as nuts and avocados, along with the use of digestive enzymes high in Lipase and Protease, omega-3 fatty acids high in DHA, magnesium, and probiotics can improve proper cholesterol levels.

Supplements for this Protocol
- JuvaTone® (for general liver support)
- Essentialzymes-4™ (for Lipase & Protease) (alternative option: Allerzyme™ or Detoxzyme®)
- Mineral Essence™ (for magnesium) (alternative option: Super Cal™ Plus or Balance Complete™ meal replacement)
- OmegaGize3™ (for DHA)
- Life 9™ (supports gut health)
- JuvaPower® (optional - for liver support)
- Daily capsule: 3 drops Lemongrass Vitality™, 2 drops Rosemary Vitality™, 1 drop Cinnamon Bark Vitality™ with 8 drops olive or avocado oil.

NOTES:

IDEAL SUPPLEMENT SCHEDULE

Before Breakfast
- Take 1 veggie capsule filled with 3 drops Lemongrass Vitality™, 2 drops Rosemary Vitality™, 1 drop Cinnamon Bark Vitality™ with 8 drops olive or avocado oil. You may pre-make a weeks worth of capsules and keep in a glass container in the refrigerator. Take with 4-8 ounces of water.

Breakfast
- Mineral Essence™ - Add 5 half-droppers (1ml each) as a shot or with juice.
- OmegaGize3™ - Take 2 capsules with breakfast.

Between Breakfast and Lunch
- JuvaTone® - Take 2 tablets

Before Lunch
- Essentialzymes-4™ - Take 2 capsules (one dual dose blister pack) before lunch.

Between Lunch and Dinner
- JuvaTone® - Take 2 tablets

Before Dinner
- Essentialzymes-4™ - Take 2 capsules (one dual dose blister pack) before dinner.

Dinner
- OmegaGize3™ - Take 2 capsules with dinner.

After Dinner
- Life 9™ - Take 1 capsule 2-3 hours after dinner, on an empty stomach. Do not take with any internal essential oils.

How long should you use this protocol?
Every person's needs are different and everyone's situation is different. Some may need to take this type of protocol every day for the rest of their lives, while others may only need it during certain seasons. Please be your own best advocate and always check with your doctor before starting or stopping any specific regimen.

These statements have not been evaluated by the Food and Drug Administration. Young Living® products are not intended to diagnose, treat, cure, or prevent any disease.

COLON CLEANSE PROTOCOL

Our intestines are home to a whole host of potential issues. Waste can pile up and depending on your age and size, you are storing anywhere from 5-20 pounds of fecal matter (poop) in your body at any given time. If not eliminated correctly, it can cause health issues. The large intestine is your colon and measures at about five feet long. The small intestine comes in at a whopping 20 feet long, making the combined length of your intestines 25 feet. Colon cleansing can improve your health by removing unwanted toxins from your gastrointestinal tract. It can improve your immune system, as well as help to improve your overall energy levels. You may take other supplements with this protocol, such as Master Formula™ and NingXia Red®.

Supplements for this Protocol
- ICP™ (laxative, intestinal tract support)
- ComforTone™ (mild laxative, intestinal tract support)
- JuvaTone® (liver support with dandelion)
- Rehemogen™ (mild laxative, intestinal tract support)
- CardioGize™ (supprots cardiovascular system)
- Digest & Cleanse™ (supports digestion)
- Essentialzyme™ (supports digestion)
- Life 9™ (supports gut health)

NOTES:

IDEAL SUPPLEMENT SCHEDULE

1 Hour Before Breakfast
- Digest & Cleanse™ - 1 capsule.

Breakfast
- CardioGize™ - Take 2 capsules just before breakfast.

Breakfast
- ICP™ - Mix 2 rounded teaspoons with at least 8 oz. of juice or water.
- ComforTone™ - Take 1 capsule.

1 Hour After Breakfast
- JuvaTone® - Take 2 tablets.

1 Hour Before Lunch
- Essentialzyme™ - Take 1 tablet.

Lunch
- Rehemogen™ - Take 3 half droppers in distilled water, just prior to lunch containing protein.
- ComforTone™ - Take 1 capsule.

1 Hour After Lunch
- JuvaTone® - Take 2 tablets.

1 Hour Before Dinner
- Digest & Cleanse™ - 1 capsule.

Dinner
- Rehemogen™ - Take 3 half droppers in distilled water just prior to dinner containing protein.
- ICP™ - Mix 2 rounded teaspoons with at least 8 oz. of juice or water.
- ComforTone™ - Take 1 capsule.

After Dinner
- Life 9™ - Take 1 capsule 2-3 hours after dinner, on an empty stomach. Do not take with any internal essential oils.

Note: Do not take CardioGize™ if you are on blood thinning medication.

How long should you use this protocol?
This is recommended as a 4-7 day protocol. Every person's needs are different and everyone's situation is different. Please be your own best advocate and always check with your doctor before starting or stopping any specific regimen.

These statements have not been evaluated by the Food and Drug Administration. Young Living® products are not intended to diagnose, treat, cure, or prevent any disease.

DIGESTIVE, GUT, AND COLON HEALTH PROTOCOL

Gut health seems to be on the top of everyone's minds. A quick look at Google trends and you will find that the search terms "best foods for gut health" had a 350% increase from 2012 to 2017 in the USA. More and more people are learning that healing our gut will go a long way in healing our various ailments. It has been studied that simply improving the gut bacteria in a patient can help support the health of diabetics, heart health, IBS, obesity, autoimmune disorders, ADHD, as well as healthy emotions and peace.

Our gut is often referred to as our little brain or second brain. The technical term for it is the enteric nervous system, or ENS. It is comprised of two thin layers that contain more than 100 million nerve cells that line your entire GI (gastrointestinal) tract, from your esophagus all the way down to your rectum. While most focus on only the intestinal tract, it is important to realize that a healthy gut starts in your mouth with your saliva enzymes.

Probiotics are the healthy or good bacteria in your gut. When you are sick, it usually means there is more bad bacteria than good bacteria. Eating foods rich in probiotics is a great way to support the healthy or good bacteria in your gut. Yogurt, kefir, and sauerkraut are excellent sources, but many people need to supplement with a broader spectrum of healthy probiotics. One of the best broad-spectrum probiotics on the market is Life 9™ from Young Living®.

Another option would be to take MightyPro™, which contains broad spectrum probiotics along with prebiotics. When you feel like the bad bacteria has overtaken the good bacteria, it is helpful to dose using Life 9™ for 1-2 days, by taking 2-6 times the recommended dose on an empty stomach, just before bed. Only do this for 1 or 2 days maximum and then resume your normal 1 capsule per day.

Supplements for this Protocol
- Life 9™ and/or MightyPro™ (probiotics)
- NingXia Red® (contains prebiotics and L-Glutamine Amino Acid)
- OmegaGize3™ (for D and omegas)
- Super B™ (supports digestion and gut health)
- AminoWise™ (contains L-Glutamine Amino Acid)
- FemiGen™ (contains Licorice Root)
- Essentialzyme™ (contains Betaine hydrochloride (HCl))

IDEAL SUPPLEMENT SCHEDULE

Breakfast
- MightyPro™ - Take one packet with breakfast.
- NingXia Red® - Drink 1-2 ounces with breakfast.
- Super B™ - Take 1 tablet with breakfast.
- OmegaGize3™ - Take 2 capsules with breakfast.
- FemiGen™ - Take 1 capsule with breakfast. (women only)

Lunch
- Super B™ - Take 1 tablet with lunch.
- OmegaGize3™ - Take 2 capsules with lunch.
- FemiGen™ - Take 1 capsule with lunch. (women only)

Between Lunch and Dinner or During Exercise
- AminoWise™ - Mix 1 scoop with 8 oz. of water and consume after lunch or during or after exercise.

Before Dinner
- Essentialzyme™ - Take 1 capsule 1 hour before dinner.

After Dinner
- Life 9™ - Take 1 capsule 2-3 hours after dinner on an empty stomach. Do not take with any internal essential oils.

How long should you use this protocol?
Every person's needs are different and everyone's situation is different. Some may need to take this type of protocol every day for the rest of their lives, while others may only need it during certain seasons. Please be your own best advocate and always check with your doctor before starting or stopping any specific regimen.

These statements have not been evaluated by the Food and Drug Administration.
Young Living® products are not intended to diagnose, treat, cure, or prevent any disease.

NOTES:

ENERGY SUPPORT PROTOCOL

We often find ourselves overworked, overwhelmed, and over everything. Energy levels drop and so does our motivation to get anything done. Supporting your digestive, immunity, and endocrine systems are important to sustained energy.

Supplements for this Protocol
- Super B™ (energy)
- EndoGize™ (ashwaganda)
- Essentialzymes-4™ (digestive enzyme)
- NingXia Red® (immunity)
- NingXia NITRO® (energy)

IDEAL SUPPLEMENT SCHEDULE

Breakfast
- NingXia Red® - Drink 1-2 ounces with breakfast.
- Super B™ - Take 1 tablet with breakfast.
- EndoGize™ - Take 1 capsule with breakfast. Use daily for four weeks. Discontinue for two weeks before resuming.

Lunch
- Essentialzymes-4™ - Take 2 capsules (one dual dose blister pack) before lunch.
- Super B™ - Take 1 tablet with lunch.
- NingXia NITRO® - Take one packet after lunch (optional)

Dinner
- Essentialzymes-4™ - Take 2 capsules (one dual dose blister pack) before dinner.
- EndoGize™ - Take 1 capsule with dinner. Use daily for four weeks. Discontinue for two weeks before resuming.

How long should you use this protocol?
Every person's needs are different and everyone's situation is different. Some may need to take this type of protocol every day for the rest of their lives, while others may only need it during certain seasons. Please be your own best advocate and always check with your doctor before starting or stopping any specific regimen.

These statements have not been evaluated by the Food and Drug Administration.
Young Living® products are not intended to diagnose, treat, cure, or prevent any disease.

NOTES:

EMOTIONAL SUPPORT PROTOCOL

Emotional states can vary drastically from day to day, moment by moment, and person to person. If you feel like your emotions are out of control, you are going through too many bouts of low or sad feelings, or you are going through hormone changes, there are several things you will want to consider. First, take a look at this list of food items that can wreak havoc on your emotions. Some you may know already, but some may be shocking. If you are dealing with sadness or are in a constant slump, this list may just change your life.

Foods to stay away from when feeling blue: gluten, soda - both regular and diet, coffee - both regular and decaf, all processed sugar, processed juice, like orange or apple juice, processed meats, like lunch meats, pepperoni, sausage, and jerky, high fructose corn syrup, energy drinks, alcohol - even wine, stay away from it, and trans fat found in frosting and many processed items. Below is a list of supplements to use to support healthy emotions. Please do not go off any medications unless you consult with your doctor. If you are taking pharmaceuticals, please do not take them at the same time as natural supplements.

Supplements for this Protocol
- OmegaGize3™ (for healthy omegas needed for the brain)
- Super B™ (for natural energy support)
- NingXia Red® (for antioxidant support)
- NingXia NITRO® (for additional energy without the fall)
- ImmuPro™ (for zinc and better sleep)
- FemiGen™ (when needed for hormonal emotions)

IDEAL SUPPLEMENT SCHEDULE

Breakfast
- NingXia Red® - Drink 1-2 ounces with breakfast.
- Super B™ - Take 1 tablet with breakfast.
- OmegaGize3™ - Take 2 capsules with breakfast.
- FemiGen™ - Take 1 capsule with breakfast. (women only)

Lunch
- Super B™ - Take 1 tablet with lunch.
- OmegaGize3™ - Take 2 capsules with lunch.
- FemiGen™ - Take 1 capsule with lunch. (women only)
- NingXia NITRO® - Take one packet after lunch. (optional)

Before Bedtime
- ImmuPro™ - Take 1-2 chewable tablets just before bed.

How long should you use this protocol?
Every person's needs are different and everyone's situation is different. Some may need to take this type of protocol every day for the rest of their lives, while others may only need it during certain seasons. Please be your own best advocate and always check with your doctor before starting or stopping any specific regimen.

These statements have not been evaluated by the Food and Drug Administration.
Young Living® products are not intended to diagnose, treat, cure, or prevent any disease.

GLUCOSE SUPPORT PROTOCOL

To help control sugar, consider the following regimen. This is for both men and women. You may continue taking other foundation nutrition supplements, if you are taking them, such as Mineral Essence™ (recommended), MultiGreens™, Life 9™, and Master Formula™. Combine this protocol with exercise and plenty of water. Drink a minimum of 10 cups of water per day. Get more fiber by adding dark leafy greens to your diet, as well as good fats, such as avocados and unsalted raw nuts. Limit red meat consumption. Limit processed carbohydrates, like pasta, bread, and foods that are high in sugar.

Supplements for this Protocol
- Balance Complete™
- NingXia Red®
- Slique® Tea - Ocotea Oolong
- Detoxzyme®
- OmegaGize3™
- Super B™
- Super Cal™ Plus
- EndoGize™

IDEAL SUPPLEMENT SCHEDULE

Breakfast
- Detoxzyme® - Take 2 capsules before breakfast.
- Balance Complete™ Shake - One shake for breakfast as a meal replacement.
- OmegaGize3™ - Take 2 capsules with breakfast.
- Super B™ - Take 1 tablet with breakfast.
- Super Cal™ Plus - Take 1 capsule with breakfast.
- NingXia Red® - Drink 1-2 ounces with breakfast.
- Slique® Tea - Ocotea Oolong - Drink 1 cup with breakfast (1 bag makes 2 cups).

Between Breakfast and Lunch
- EndoGize™ - Take 1 capsule between breakfast and lunch.

Lunch
- Detoxzyme® - Take 2 capsules before lunch.
- OmegaGize3™ - Take 2 capsules with lunch.
- Super B™ - Take 1 tablet the with lunch.
- Super Cal™ Plus - Take 1 capsule with lunch.
- Slique® Tea - Ocotea Oolong - Drink 1 cup with lunch (1 bag makes 2 cups).

Between Lunch and Dinner
- EndoGize™ - Take 1 capsule between lunch and dinner.

Dinner
- Detoxzyme® - Take 2 capsules before dinner.
- OmegaGize3™ - Take 2 capsules with dinner.

How long should you use this protocol?
Every person's needs are different and everyone's situation is different. Some may need to take this type of protocol every day for the rest of their lives, while others may only need it during certain seasons. Please be your own best advocate and always check with your doctor before starting or stopping any specific regimen.

These statements have not been evaluated by the Food and Drug Administration. Young Living® products are not intended to diagnose, treat, cure, or prevent any disease.

GLUTEN SUPPORT PROTOCOL

Gluten sensitivity and intolerance in the form of Celiac Disease can vary greatly from person to person. Celiac Disease presents in various forms from bloating and gas to severe stomach cramping and pain that can last for a day or two. Gluten allergies or sensitivities can vary from headaches, swelling, bloating, gas, acne, and even intense bouts of emotional instability from anger to extreme sadness.

Many people have sensitivities to gluten and may not know it. The only real way to find relief is to not consume any gluten. Gluten is found in anything containing American grain wheat, barley grass, and rye. It turns up in soy sauce, salad dressings, and even french fries that have been fried in oil that was previously used for something such as battered onion rings.

People with gluten intolerances absolutely must check every label and take extra precautions when eating out. Even the smallest particle will cause a response. The following protocol is not meant to help you eat gluten. It is a means to help your body process it through your system if you are eating something that could have cross contamination. This usually happens when eating at a friend's home or out at a restaurant. Digestive enzymes are a key support to help your body digest gluten.

Supplements for this Protocol
- Essentialzymes-4™
- Detoxzyme®

IDEAL SUPPLEMENT SCHEDULE

Take 10 minutes before eating a meal that may contain gluten
- Essentialzymes-4™ - Take 2 capsules (one dual dose blister pack).
- Detoxzyme® - Take 2-4 capsules.

How long should you use this protocol?
Every person's needs are different and everyone's situation is different. Some may need to take this type of protocol every day for the rest of their lives, while others may only need it during certain seasons. Please be your own best advocate and always check with your doctor before starting or stopping any specific regimen.

These statements have not been evaluated by the Food and Drug Administration.
Young Living® products are not intended to diagnose, treat, cure, or prevent any disease.

NOTES:

HAIR, SKIN, AND NAILS PROTOCOL

Having great hair, skin, and nails is something women strive for. Men too, but women especially. The three keys to a healthy integumentary system are: a diet rich in a colorful array of veggies, drink lots of water, and find daily peace. Stress is one of the most prevalent causes of hair loss, brittle nails, and skin conditions such as rashes and blemishes. One of the best things you can do for your integumentary system is to relax, and drink a tall glass of water. Taking a walk daily that gets your heart pumping and skin sweating is helpful too, in order to stimulate your circulatory system and lymphatic system which is needed to help flush toxins from your skin.

The most common supplements to support the largest organ in the body, also known as the integumentary system (your hair, skin, nails, and exocrine glands), are antioxidants in the form of vitamins A, C, and E, Coenzyme Q10, fatty acids found in fish oils, all the B vitamins, D3, K2, calcium, MSM, magnesium, and small amounts of selenium.

Supplements for this Protocol
- Sulfurzyme™ (MSM to strengthen hair and nails)
- AgilEase™ (collagen for glowing skin)
- NingXia Red® (antioxidant)
- OmegaGize3™ (Vitamin D3 for hair loss, Coenzyme Q10 for free radicals, and EPA for wrinkles and acne)
- Super Cal™ Plus (calcium for hair loss, magnesium for wrinkles and strong nails, D3 for hair, K2 for aging and skin)
- Super C™ Chewables and Tablets (antioxidant)
- Super B™ (a must for glowing skin and strong nails)
- Mineral Essence™ (magnesium for wrinkles and strong nails, selenium for hair)

NOTES:

IDEAL SUPPLEMENT SCHEDULE

Breakfast
- Super C™ - Take 1-2 tablets before breakfast.
- NingXia Red® - Drink 1-2 ounces with breakfast.
- OmegaGize3™ - Take 2 capsules with breakfast.
- Super Cal™ Plus - Take 2 capsules with breakfast.
- Super B™ - Take 1 tablet with breakfast.
- Mineral Essence™ - Take 5 half-droppers (1 ml each) with breakfast. You may use five 00 veggie capsules.

Between Breakfast and Lunch
- Sulfurzyme™ - Take 2 capsules or 1/2 teaspoon powder with juice or water.

Lunch
- OmegaGize3™ - Take 2 capsules with lunch.
- AgilEase™ - Take 2 capsules with lunch.
- Super B™ - Take 1 tablet with lunch.
- Super C™ Chewable - Take 1 chewable tablet with lunch.

Between Lunch and Dinner
- Sulfurzyme™ - Take 2 capsules or 1/2 teaspoon powder with juice or water.

Dinner
- Mineral Essence™ - Take 5 half-droppers (1 ml each) with dinner. You may use five 00 veggie capsules.
- Super C™ Chewable - Take 1 chewable tablet with dinner.

How long should you use this protocol?
Every person's needs are different and everyone's situation is different. Some may need to take this type of protocol every day for the rest of their lives, while others may only need it during certain seasons. Please be your own best advocate and always check with your doctor before starting or stopping any specific regimen.

These statements have not been evaluated by the Food and Drug Administration. Young Living® products are not intended to diagnose, treat, cure, or prevent any disease.

NOTES:

HORMONE SUPPORT PROTOCOLS INTRODUCTION

Our hormones come from our endocrine system. It is comprised of 10 glands, nine for each sex. The eight glands common to both sexes are the hypothalamus, pineal, pituitary, thyroid, parathyroid, thymus, adrenals, and pancreas. For men, they also have testes, and for women, ovaries.

These glands secrete various hormones into the body using the bloodstream to help the body maintain homeostasis or balance within the body systems. The hormones support how we grow and develop, our metabolism and energy levels, our stress response, our wake and sleep patterns, the reproductive systems, and a whole host of other functions. It is important to have healthy blood and a healthy supply of that blood since the blood is the carrier of all the hormones.

There are four outside factors that can drastically affect your hormones positively or negatively. These factors are stress levels, sleep patterns, diet, and exercise habits. If you are experiencing changes in your hormones, consider these simple (or possibly not so simple) modifications to your lifestyle to support the needs of your body. Work on one or two at a time over the course of 30 days. Once you feel good about that change, try tackling another one for the next 30 days. Monitor how you feel and any positive changes you see.

1. **Drink more water.** Upping your water consumption will help your circulation and improve not only your blood flow but also your ability to remove waste from your body. Try to get half your body weight in ounces of water. As an example, if you are 200 lbs, you need 100 oz of water. If you are 150 lbs, you need 75 oz of water.

2. **Add greens.** Add 1-2 more servings of dark green veggies or leafy greens. This will help rid your body of oxidative stress and will help your blood and hormones work better. We are supposed to get at least 3-4 servings of vegetables per day, but many of us are way under that.

3. **Get more sleep.** Go to bed one hour earlier than normal. Sleep is such an important factor when supporting your hormones. When you are sleep deprived (less than seven hours of sleep per night) your hormones become uncoordinated. Here are a couple reasons to get more sleep if you still aren't convinced: #1 - Lack of sleep increases your hunger hormone, so when you are awake, your brain will tell you to eat more, even if you don't need to and #2 - Lack of sleep causes your fat storage to get out of whack. Not getting enough sleep increases insulin resistance, essentially contributing to weight gain and obesity.

4. **Go on a walk.** Walking increases oxygen to your blood and brain, which is paramount for hormones to travel where they need to go. It is like traveling on a winding dirt road as opposed to a freshly paved straight highway. Try to take a 15-30 minute walk at least five times a week.

5. **Create space.** We tend to say "yes" to too many things. Start saying no, and create more white space on your calendar and your daily to-do list. This will give you some much needed downtime. Every time someone asks you to do something, consider if it is the best thing for you to do. Not every need is a calling. It is important to not overwhelm yourself helping everyone but you.

6. **Take a nap.** If you have an overwhelming amount of items on your to-do list, you may feel guilty taking a nap. Don't worry about what others might think. Just do it. Taking a 30 minute nap, or even a 10 minute power nap if you are able to, will help your energy levels and motivation throughout the day. Because sleep is important to hormone production, a nap will give your body a quick refueling.

7. **Limit noise.** While social media has allowed us to seemingly get a lot more done and stay connected to a lot more people, it has also very successfully added loads of stress to our lives. Stress from social media comes from many angles: FOMO (fear of missing out), keeping up with the Joneses, people-pleasing, and time-sucking. It is the ultimate distraction and the ultimate relationship blocker. Next time you go to a restaurant, take a look around. Most parties are all on their cell phones. I recommend leaving your phone in the car when you are eating out, or leave your cell phone in the kitchen when you go to bed. Having a cell phone in your bedroom can damage your sleep patterns because of the incessant need to check it, but also because of the electro-magnetic radiation that emits from cell phones that is poisoning your ability to sleep soundly. If you need your phone in your bedroom, simply shut the entire thing down at a specific time, at least one hour before bedtime.

8. **Limit coffee and alcohol.** Coffee and alcohol are both endocrine disruptors. This means they mess with your hormones. Coffee tells your adrenal glands that they can take a break. You've got it covered so the adrenals do not need to produce any "wake up" hormone (cortisol). Even one cup is damaging to your endocrine system. Alcohol dumps massive amounts of sugar into your system. Alcohol also imposes damaging effects on growth, metabolism, energy storage, bones, blood pressure, and the ability to get pregnant (this goes for both sperm count in men, and ovulation in women).

9. **Ditch white sugar.** Sugar in the form of table sugar and refined carbohydrates, such as bread and pasta, are a major insulin hormone disruptor. Insulin is a highly connected hormone to all the other hormones and can directly affect a woman's estrogen levels and a man's testosterone levels. It is one of the hardest things to do, but going on a sugar moratorium for 30 days, and then hopefully longer, will go a long way in supporting healthy hormones. A sugar moratorium (aka no sugar, aka death to sugar) means not eating processed sugar. You will want to stay away from items with high glycemic indexes such as bread, muffins, cookies, and anything containing white sugar and/or wheat.

10. **Limit junk.** Both fast food and processed food contain hormone disrupting ingredients in the form of GMOs, preservatives, additives, synthetic flavoring, and other nasty things. Processed foods are notorious for messing with our bodies. A simple trip to any country outside of the USA, that has not adopted USA food practices, and you will find a much healthier nation with far less obesity, heart disease, and osteoporosis. Start by changing one meal that is usually processed or from a fast food establishment to a meal that is made with real ingredients. Some sneaky forms of processed foods to stay away from are: sandwiches, any processed meats such as sausage, pepperoni, and deli meats, milk (unless you live on a farm, do not consume processed milk), store-bought orange juice, sports drinks (while these seem like they replenish your body, all they are doing is flooding your system with sugar and salt), and bacon. Bacon? Noooooo! OK I hear you, but seriously, bacon is one of the worst foods you can eat. That is unless, of course, you own some pigs and are able to make your own. Otherwise, most bacon is filled with preservatives, nitrates, and hormones that you do NOT want in your system. Visit www.endo180.com for more tips on resetting your endocrine system through your diet.

11. **Ditch and switch.** Ditch and switch. Get rid of all the synthetic products in your home and replace them with synthetic-free versions. Petrochemicals are considered the worst invader on your endocrine system. They make up the majority of the plastics and synthetic molecules in many of the household and personal care products on the market today. Consider all areas such as cleaning supplies, laundry detergent, fabric softener, dish washing detergent, air fresheners, candles, facial wash and lotions, body lotions, toothpaste, deodorant, makeup, hand soap, hand sanitizer, shampoo, conditioner, body wash, etc.

While making lifestyle changes takes time, and in some cases can be next to impossible, because, you know, we are, after all, only human, I encourage you to consider adding some healthful supplements to your daily regimen. The following protocols cover various hormone needs. You will find five protocols: general hormone health for women, general hormone health for men, menopause and fertility support, adrenal support, and thyroid support.

NOTES:

HORMONE HEALTH GENERAL (WOMEN) PROTOCOL

The below protocol is for general hormone health in women. It is important to monitor yourself to see how you feel. You can start this protocol by only doing the "breakfast" capsules for two weeks, then add the "lunch" capsules. Take note of how you feel and what amount works best for your needs.

Supplements for this Protocol
- PD 80/20™
- FemiGen™
- OmegaGize3™

IDEAL SUPPLEMENT SCHEDULE

Breakfast
- OmegaGize3™ - Take 2 capsules with breakfast.
- FemiGen™ - Take 1 capsule with breakfast.
- PD 80/20™ - Take 1 capsule with breakfast.

Lunch
- FemiGen™ - Take 1 capsule with lunch.
- OmegaGize3™ - Take 2 capsules with lunch.

How long should you use this protocol?
Every person's needs are different and everyone's situation is different. Some may need to take this type of protocol every day for the rest of their lives, while others may only need it during certain seasons. Please be your own best advocate and always check with your doctor before starting or stopping any specific regimen.

These statements have not been evaluated by the Food and Drug Administration. Young Living® products are not intended to diagnose, treat, cure, or prevent any disease.

NOTES:

HORMONE HEALTH GENERAL (MEN) PROTOCOL

The below protocol is for general hormone health for men. It is important to monitor yourself to see how you feel. Note: While EndoGize™ states it is a women's supplement, that is only because the majority of customers in Young Living® are women. Please refer to the write up on EndoGize™ and you will see how powerful this supplement is for men specifically.

Supplements for this Protocol
- EndoGize™
- Prostate Health™ (optional)
- OmegaGize3™ (D3, Omegas)
- PowerGize™ (Fenugreek)
- JuvaPower™ (Ginger root)

IDEAL SUPPLEMENT SCHEDULE

Breakfast
- EndoGize™ - Take 1 capsule with breakfast. Use daily for four weeks. Discontinue for two weeks before resuming.
- OmegaGize3™ - Take 2 capsules with breakfast.
- JuvaPower™ - Sprinkle 1 tbsp onto food, mix into smoothie or 4 oz of water.

Between Breakfast and Lunch
- Prostate Health™ (optional) - Take 1 capsule between meals.

Lunch
- PowerGize™ - Take 2 capsules with lunch.
- JuvaPower™ - Sprinkle 1 tbsp onto food, mix into smoothie or 4 oz of water.

Between Lunch and Dinner
- Prostate Health™ (optional) - Take 1 capsule between meals.

Dinner
- EndoGize™ - Take 1 capsule with dinner. Use daily for four weeks. Discontinue for two weeks before resuming.
- OmegaGize3™ - Take 2 capsules with dinner.
- JuvaPower™ - Sprinkle 1 tbsp onto food, mix into smoothie or 4 oz of water.

How long should you use this protocol?
EndoGize™ should be used daily for four weeks. Discontinue for two weeks before resuming. For the whole protocol, every person's needs are different and everyone's situation is different. Some may need to take this protocol every day for the rest of their lives, while others may only need it during certain seasons. Please be your own best advocate and always check with your doctor before starting or stopping any specific regimen.

These statements have not been evaluated by the Food and Drug Administration. Young Living® products are not intended to diagnose, treat, cure, or prevent any disease.

HORMONE HEALTH - ADRENAL SUPPORT PROTOCOL

The adrenal glands are a part of your endocrine system, that regulates energy output in the form of adrenaline and cortisol. When you are stressed out or get scared, your adrenals release hormones to help get you through the experience. It is commonly referred to as the "fight or flight" response. When you go through long periods of heightened stress, your body will produce more cortisol and adrenaline than normal for an extended period. This effectively wears out your adrenals and this could lead to what is called adrenal fatigue.

This protocol is not a treatment for adrenal fatigue. It is meant to help you manage stressful seasons so you do not get to the point of adrenal fatigue. If you are planning a move, switching careers, working through grief and loss, or anything that you know would cause longer periods of stress, you will want to consider this protocol. It is also important to protect your cells during times of stress by reducing the amount of processed sugar and raising the amount of water you consume. Also, try to get 1-2 hours of extra sleep. While this may sound impossible during stressful times of your life, it is better to get some extra sleep than to binge watch television.

There are two different supplements to choose from. CortiStop™ would be selected when you are under mild stress, and EndoGize™ would be selected when you are under severe stress. Please note: EndoGize™ is only to be taken daily for four weeks and then you must discontinue for two weeks before resuming. Mineral Essence™ may be taken once or twice a day. Super B™ may be taken as one dose of 2 tablets with breakfast, but it is recommended to space out the 2 tablets for more prolonged energy support benefits. Super C™ is a completely different supplement compared to Super C™ Chewables. Super C™ regular tablets are the ones you want for this protocol.

Supplements for this Protocol
- CortiStop™ (mild)
- EndoGize™ (severe)
- Super B™
- Super C™
- Mineral Essence™ (for needed magnesium)

NOTE: There are two protocols to consider. One uses CortiStop™ and one uses EndoGize™. Please see individual supplement write-ups to determine which is right for your needs.

IDEAL SUPPLEMENT SCHEDULE USING CORTISTOP™

Before Breakfast
- Super C™ - Take 1-2 tablets before breakfast.
- CortiStop™ - Take 1-2 capsules before breakfast.

Breakfast
- Super B™ - Take 1 tablet with breakfast.
- Mineral Essence™ - Take 5 half-droppers (1 ml each) with breakfast. You may use five 00 veggie capsules.

Lunch
- Super B™ - Take 1 tablet with lunch.
- Mineral Essence™ - Take 5 half-droppers (1 ml each) with dinner. You may use five 00 veggie capsules.

Before Bedtime
- CortiStop™ - Take 1-2 capsules before bedtime.

IDEAL SUPPLEMENT SCHEDULE USING ENDOGIZE™

Before Breakfast
- Super C™ - Take 1-2 tablets before breakfast.

Breakfast
- EndoGize™ - Take 1 capsule with breakfast. Use daily for four weeks. Discontinue for two weeks before resuming.
- Super B™ - Take 1 tablet with breakfast.
- Mineral Essence™ - Take 5 half-droppers (1 ml each) with breakfast. You may use five 00 veggie capsules.

Lunch
- Super B™ - Take 1 tablet with lunch.

Dinner
- EndoGize™ - Take 1 capsule with dinner. Use daily for four weeks. Discontinue for two weeks before resuming.
- Mineral Essence™ - Take 5 half-droppers (1 ml each) with dinner. You may use five 00 veggie capsules.

How long should you use this protocol?
EndoGize™ should be used daily for four weeks. Discontinue for two weeks before resuming. For the whole protocol, every person's needs are different and everyone's situation is different. Some may need to take this protocol every day for the rest of their lives, while others may only need it during certain seasons. Please be your own best advocate and always check with your doctor before starting or stopping any specific regimen.

These statements have not been evaluated by the Food and Drug Administration. Young Living® products are not intended to diagnose, treat, cure, or prevent any disease.

HORMONE HEALTH (WOMEN) - MENOPAUSE & FERTILITY SUPPORT PROTOCOL

As we age, our hormone production changes. We still have and need our hormones, but in some areas, such as reproduction, these hormones are not as necessary. This shift in hormones can cause undesirable effects in our body, such as night sweats, temperature regulation from hot to cold, and erratic mood swings. The supplements in this protocol will help regulate this process.

It is important to note, women who are desiring to get pregnant may also follow this protocol. If you are going through menopause, and do not wish to become pregnant, please use precautions. This protocol effectively regulates and restores your reproductive system. During menopause, this protocol will slow down the process, and you could get pregnant. During normal reproductive years, this protocol will support a healthy system.

If you are trying to get pregnant, the #1 factor that was already discussed needs to be highlighted again here. You must, and I mean MUST, remove all synthetic toxins from your surroundings to the very best of your ability. Get rid of all the synthetic products in your home and workspace and replace them with synthetic-free versions.

Petrochemicals are considered the worst invader on your endocrine system and can block you from getting pregnant. They can also hinder sperm count, how fast they swim, and their DNA validity. Petrochemicals make up the majority of the plastics and synthetic molecules in many of the household and personal care products on the market today.

Consider all areas such as cleaning supplies, laundry detergent, fabric softener, dishwashing detergent, air fresheners, candles, facial wash and lotions, body lotions, toothpaste, deodorant, makeup, hand soap, hand sanitizer, shampoo, conditioner, body wash, etc.

Try to remove actual plastics as well. Memory foam is a massive petrochemical and should be avoided. Memory foam is found in many mattresses, pillows, running and walking shoes, and other items. Plastic shower curtains and pool blow up toys should not be used. If you can smell the plastic, that is the bad kind. Consider eliminating plastic water bottles and opt for using filtered water that you drink out of glass or stainless steel.

Supplements for this Protocol
- Progessence Plus™
- FemiGen™
- Master Formula™ (vitamins A, B, D, E)

IDEAL SUPPLEMENT SCHEDULE

Before Breakfast
- Progessence Plus™ - Rub 1 drop on each inner arm, from the inner elbow to the inner wrist, when you wake up. You may rotate application sites. Other areas to apply: back of neck, front of neck, on the bottom of your feet, or on your inner thighs.

Breakfast
- FemiGen™ - Take 1 capsule with breakfast.
- Master Formula™ - Take full packet with breakfast.

Lunch
- FemiGen™ - Take 1 capsule with lunch.

Before Bedtime
- Progessence Plus™ - Rub 1 drop on each inner arm, from the inner elbow to the inner wrist, in the evening before you go to sleep. You may rotate application sites. Other areas to apply: back of neck, front of neck, on the bottom of your feet, or on your inner thighs.

How long should you use this protocol?
Every person's needs are different and everyone's situation is different. Some may need to take this type of protocol every day for the rest of their lives, while others may only need it during certain seasons. Please be your own best advocate and always check with your doctor before starting or stopping any specific regimen.

These statements have not been evaluated by the Food and Drug Administration.
Young Living® products are not intended to diagnose, treat, cure, or prevent any disease.

NOTES:

HORMONE HEALTH - THYROID SUPPORT PROTOCOL

Supporting your thyroid can help increase energy, improve digestion and metabolism, help with mood swings, and bone health. It is important to consider dietary changes as well, like eating more veggies and going on a daily walk to increase circulation. Please consult your doctor if you are currently on a thyroid supporting regimen. It is best to bring in the labels for each of the below supplements so he or she can see what they contain.

Supplements for this Protocol
- Thyromin™ (natural thyroid support with pig and cow gland extracts)
- MultiGreens™ (contains eleuthero to support the thyroid)
- JuvaTone™ (contains echinacea to support the thyroid)

IDEAL SUPPLEMENT SCHEDULE

Between Breakfast and Lunch
- JuvaTone® - Take 2 tablets between meals.

Lunch
- MultiGreens™ - Take 3 capsules with lunch.

Between Lunch and Dinner
- JuvaTone® - Take 2 tablets between meals.

Dinner
- MultiGreens™ - Take 3 capsules with dinner.

Before Bedtime
- Thyromin™ - Take 1-2 capsules, just before bed, on an empty stomach.

How long should you use this protocol?
Every person's needs are different and everyone's situation is different. Some may need to take this type of protocol every day for the rest of their lives, while others may only need it during certain seasons. Please be your own best advocate and always check with your doctor before starting or stopping any specific regimen.

These statements have not been evaluated by the Food and Drug Administration. Young Living® products are not intended to diagnose, treat, cure, or prevent any disease.

IMMUNITY SUPPORT PROTOCOL

When you ask a doctor, "What is the most important function in our body?" They will tell you that your immunity is the thing to keep strong. Our immunity is supported by our blood, lymph nodes, and gut. Supplements high in antioxidants are a must, but also a good diet, exercise, and getting enough sleep are important in supporting your immunity. The following is recommended to support all areas of your immunity. You may add additional supplements to this protocol, such as Super Cal™ Plus, Super B™, and Essentialzymes-4™, or any that you are already taking.

Supplements for this Protocol
- NingXia Red®
- Super C™ Tablets
- Super C™ Chewables
- Inner Defense™
- Life 9™
- ImmuPro™

NOTE: Both Super C™ supplements are needed for this protocol. They are not the same.

IDEAL SUPPLEMENT SCHEDULE

Before Breakfast
- Inner Defense™ - Take 1 capsule when you wake up, at least 20 minutes before breakfast.

Breakfast
- NingXia Red® - Drink 1-2 ounces with breakfast.
- Super C™ - Take 1-2 tablets before breakfast.

Lunch
- NingXia Red® - Drink 1-2 ounces with lunch or in the afternoon.

Dinner
- Super C™ Chewable - Take 1 chewable tablet with dinner.

After Dinner
- Life 9™ - Take 1 capsule 2-3 hours after dinner, on an empty stomach. Do not take with any internal essential oils.
- ImmuPro™ - Take 1 chewable tablet 30 minutes before bed and at least an hour after taking Life 9™.

How long should you use this protocol?
Every person's needs are different and everyone's situation is different. Some may need to take this type of protocol every day for the rest of their lives, while others may only need it during certain seasons. Please be your own best advocate and always check with your doctor before starting or stopping any specific regimen.

JOINT AND MOBILITY HEALTH PROTOCOL

As we age our mobility declines. Our connective tissue is not as strong and our joints can become inflamed. This is also true of athletes who are putting extra pressure and continual strain on the joints. For those of you who are not aggressive athletes, it is always recommended to stretch every day as well as get a minimum of 30 minutes of exercise per day. A walk around the block can sometimes be the best remedy. This will get your lymphatic and circulatory systems moving, to help rid waste and oxygenate your cells.

It is important to also drink plenty of water when desiring the support of healthy joints, ligaments, bones, and muscles. Simply drink half your body weight number in ounces. For example: if you are 200 pounds, you would strive to drink 100 ounces of water per day.

Another often misunderstood area of concern, when it comes to joint and mobility health, is our diet. Many foods can cause inflammation in our bodies and the removal of these items can help tremendously. Consider lowering the intake of, or eliminating altogether processed meats (sliced sandwich meats or canned meats), gluten (anything containing flour, such as breads and pasta), soybean and vegetable oils, processed foods such as chips and crackers, sodas, sugary drinks such as alcohol, trans fats found in fried foods, dairy such as cheese and milk, aspartame (sugar substitute), and all items containing corn such as popcorn, chips, corn tortillas, many cereals, and items where corn is hiding, such as salad dressings, chewing gum, peanut butter, soft drink sweeteners (corn syrup). To find a great meal plan head to www.endo180.com to help you take charge of the inflammatory response in your body. If you have a hard time with food elimination, please consider taking a digestive enzyme. The one recommended below is Allerzyme™.

Supplementation can help support in many ways. Using products with MSM, turmeric, omega-3 fatty acids, and spirulina may help improve mobility in both athletes and people who need additional support. It is also important to support your overall immunity and gut health.

Supplements for this Protocol
- Life 9™ and/or MightyPro™
- NingXia Red®
- OmegaGize3™
- Sulfurzyme™ (capsules or powder drink mix)
- AgilEase™
- MultiGreens™
- Allerzyme™ (optional)

IDEAL SUPPLEMENT SCHEDULE

Breakfast
- Allerzyme™ (optional) - Take 1 capsule just prior to breakfast.
- MightyPro™ - Take 1 packet with breakfast.
- NingXia Red® - Drink 1-2 ounces with breakfast.
- OmegaGize3™ - Take 2 capsules with breakfast.
- AgilEase™ - Take 2 capsules with breakfast.

Between Breakfast and Lunch
- Sulfurzyme™ - Take 2 capsules or 1/2 tsp powder with juice or water.

Lunch
- Allerzyme™ (optional) - Take 1 capsule just prior to lunch.
- OmegaGize3™ - Take 2 capsules with lunch.
- MultiGreens™ - Take 3 capsules with lunch.

Between Lunch and Dinner
- Sulfurzyme™ - Take 2 capsules or 1/2 tsp powder with juice or water.

Dinner
- Allerzyme™ (optional) - Take 1 capsule just prior to dinner.
- MultiGreens™ - Take 3 capsules with dinner.

After Dinner
- Life 9™ - Take 1 capsule, 2-3 hours after dinner, on an empty stomach.
- Do not take with any internal essential oils.

How long should you use this protocol?
Every person's needs are different and everyone's situation is different. Some may need to take this type of protocol every day for the rest of their lives, while others may only need it during certain seasons. Please be your own best advocate and always check with your doctor before starting or stopping any specific regimen.

These statements have not been evaluated by the Food and Drug Administration.
Young Living® products are not intended to diagnose, treat, cure, or prevent any disease.

NOTES:

LIVER SUPPORT PROTOCOL

The liver is about the size of a football and sits on the right side of the belly inside the ribcage. It filters blood from the digestive system. It is the detox center of your body. Support your liver by eating a healthy diet high in vegetables and fiber, exercise regularly, don't drink alcohol that often, and try to avoid synthetics in the form of processed foods. The supplements in this protocol are used for general liver support.

Supplements for this Protocol
- AgilEase™ (turmeric is a powerful liver detoxifier)
- JuvaTone® (for overall liver support with high protein diets)
- JuvaPower™ (for general liver and intestine support)
- Juva Cleanse™ Vitality™ capsule (supports liver)
- JuvaFlex™ Vitality™ capsule (supports liver and digestion)
- GLF™ Vitality™ capsule (supports gallbladder and liver)

IDEAL SUPPLEMENT SCHEDULE

Before Breakfast
- Juva Cleanse™ Vitality™ - Add 2 drops Juva Cleanse Vitality™ to a veggie capsule, top off with grapeseed or olive oil, and take with 8 oz of water.

Breakfast
- JuvaPower™ - Sprinkle 1 tbsp onto food, mix into smoothie or 4 oz of water.
- AgilEase™ - Take 2 capsules with breakfast.

Between Breakfast and Lunch
- JuvaTone® - Take 2 tablets between meals.

Lunch
- JuvaPower™ - Sprinkle 1 tbsp onto food, mix into smoothie or 4 oz of water.
- JuvaFlex™ Vitality™ - Add 2 drops JuvaFlex Vitality™ to a veggie capsule, top off with grapeseed or olive oil, and take with at least 8 oz of water.

Between Lunch and Dinner
- JuvaTone® - Take 2 tablets between meals.

Dinner
- JuvaPower™ - Sprinkle 1 tbsp onto food, mix into smoothie or 4 oz of water.

Before Bedtime
- GLF™ Vitality™ - Add 2 drops GLF Vitality™ to a veggie capsule, top off with grapeseed or olive oil, and take with at least 8 ounces of water.

How long should you use this protocol?
Take this for a 3-4 day liver support or for up to one month. This is not recommended for 365 day use. Every person's needs are different and everyone's situation is different. Some may need to take this type of protocol every day for the rest of their lives, while others may only need it during certain seasons. Please be your own best advocate and always check with your doctor before starting or stopping any specific regimen.

These statements have not been evaluated by the Food and Drug Administration. Young Living® products are not intended to diagnose, treat, cure, or prevent any disease.

STRESS & SLEEP SUPPORT PROTOCOL

When you are not getting enough sleep, your response to stress gets compromised. When you are stressed out, your ability to sleep well gets compromised. It is a terrible lose-lose cycle. Most people need 7-9 hours of sleep per night, and the average American gets 6.8 hours of sleep. Over time, this will compound upon itself, causing sleep deprivation. Sleep deprivation causes memory loss and a slower functionality rate in motor skills. Lack of sleep increases your hunger hormone, so when you are awake, your brain will tell you to eat more, even if you don't need to. Lack of sleep also causes your fat storage to get out of whack. Not getting enough sleep increases insulin resistance, essentially contributing to weight gain and obesity. Here are some supplements that may help you get a more restful night's sleep.

Supplements for this Protocol
- Super B™ (for stress)
- Mineral Essence™ (for magnesium)
- CardioGize™ (for resilience)
- ImmuPro™ (for melatonin and immunity)
- Sleep Essence™ (for melatonin and immunity)

IDEAL SUPPLEMENT SCHEDULE

Breakfast
- CardioGize™ - Take 2 capsules before breakfast.
- Super B™ - Take 1 tablet with breakfast.
- Mineral Essence™ - Take 5 half-droppers (1 ml each) with breakfast. You may use five 00 veggie capsules.

Lunch
- Super B™ - Take 1 tablet with lunch.

Dinner
- Mineral Essence™ - Take 5 half-droppers (1 ml each) with dinner. You may use five 00 veggie capsules.

Before Bedtime
- ImmuPro™ - Take 1-2 chewable tablets just before bed.
- Sleep Essence™- Take 1-2 capsules just before bed.

How long should you use this protocol?
Every person's needs are different and everyone's situation is different. Some may need to take this type of protocol every day for the rest of their lives, while others may only need it during certain seasons. Please be your own best advocate and always check with your doctor before starting or stopping any specific regimen.

These statements have not been evaluated by the Food and Drug Administration. Young Living® products are not intended to diagnose, treat, cure, or prevent any disease.

URINARY SUPPORT PROTOCOL

The urinary system, or renal system, is made up of the kidneys, ureters, bladder, and the urethra. It is important to support your urinary system by drinking lots of fluids. Water is best, and it is recommended that you get at least 80-100 ounces of water per day; more if you are excessively sweating or exercising.

Supplements for this Protocol
- K & B™
- CardioGize™
- ComforTone™
- Super C™ Tablets
- NingXia Red®

IDEAL SUPPLEMENT SCHEDULE

Before Breakfast
- CardioGize™ - Take 2 capsules.
- Super C™ - Take 1-2 tablets.

Breakfast
- K & B™ - Take 3 half droppers in distilled water.
- NingXia Red® - Drink 1-2 ounces with breakfast.
- ComforTone™ - Take 1 capsule.

Lunch
- K & B™ - Take 3 half droppers in distilled water.

Between Lunch and Dinner
- JuvaTone® - Take 2 tablets between meals.

Dinner
- K & B™ - Take 3 half droppers in distilled water.
- ComforTone™ - Take 1 capsule.

Note: Do not take CardioGize™ if you are on blood thinning medication.

How long should you use this protocol?
Every person's needs are different and everyone's situation is different. Some may need to take this type of protocol every day for the rest of their lives, while others may only need it during certain seasons. Please be your own best advocate and always check with your doctor before starting or stopping any specific regimen.

These statements have not been evaluated by the Food and Drug Administration. Young Living® products are not intended to diagnose, treat, cure, or prevent any disease.

WEIGHT SUPPORT PROTOCOL

Maintaining a healthy weight becomes more challenging as we grow older and our metabolism slows down. This protocol works well when you combine it with healthy eating and a daily exercise routine.

Supplements for this Protocol
- Slique® Shake
- Slique® CitraSlim
- Slique® Tea
- Slique® Bars
- Slique® Chewing Gum
- Peppermint, Lemon, Grapefruit , and Thieves® Vitality™

IDEAL SUPPLEMENT SCHEDULE

Before Breakfast
- Slique® CitraSlim™ - Take 2 powder capsules with 8 ounces of water.

Breakfast
- Slique® Shake - Drink one as a meal replacement for breakfast.
- Slique® Tea - Drink and add 1 drop of Thieves® Vitality™.

Between Breakfast and Lunch
- Infused Water - Drink one 20+ ounce water with 1 drop Peppermint Vitality™ and 1-2 drops each of Lemon Vitality™ and Grapefruit Vitality™.
- Slique® Bar - Eat one as a snack.

Lunch
- Eat a sensible, healthy lunch.

Between Lunch and Dinner
- Slique® CitraSlim™ - Take 1 powder capsule and 1 Slique® CitraSlim liquid capsule in the afternoon before 3pm.
- Infused Water - Drink one 20+ ounce water with 1 drop Peppermint Vitality™ and 1-2 drops each of Lemon Vitality™ and Grapefruit Vitality™.
- Slique® Tea - Drink in the afternoon.
- Eat a healthy snack or one Slique® Bar.
- Slique® gum - Chew 1 tablet to help hunger cravings.

Dinner
- Eat a sensible healthy dinner.

Exercise
- Get in a minimum of five 30-minute walks per week.

How long should you use this protocol?
30-90 days at a time. Every person's needs are different and everyone's situation is different. Some may need to take this type of protocol every day for the rest of their lives, while others may only need it during certain seasons. Please be your own best advocate and always check with your doctor before starting or stopping any specific regimen.

These statements have not been evaluated by the Food and Drug Administration.
Young Living® products are not intended to diagnose, treat, cure, or prevent any disease.

KID'S HEALTH PROTOCOL - GENERAL HEALTH SUPPORT

For kids 4 years and older

Supplements for this Protocol
- NingXia Red® (immunity support)
- KidScents® MightyZyme™ (digestive enzymes)
- KidScents® MightyVites™ (full-spectrum vitamin)
- KidScents® MightyPro™ (prebiotics and probiotics)
- Super C™ Chewables (antioxidants and immunity support)

IDEAL SUPPLEMENT SCHEDULE

Breakfast
- KidScents® MightyVites™ - Take 2 chewable tablets.
- KidScents® MightyZyme™ - Take 1 chewable tablet.
- KidScents® MightyPro™ - Take 1 sachet.
- Super C™ Chewables - Take 1 chewable tablet.
- Drink 1-2 ounces of NingXia Red®.

Dinner
- KidScents® MightyVites™ - Take 2 chewable tablets.
- KidScents® MightyZyme™ - Take 1 chewable tablet.
- Super C™ Chewables - Take 1 chewable tablet.

How long should you use this protocol?
Every person's needs are different and everyone's situation is different. Some may need to take this type of protocol every day for the rest of their lives, while others may only need it during certain seasons. Please be your child's best advocate and always check with your doctor before starting or stopping any specific regimen.

These statements have not been evaluated by the Food and Drug Administration. Young Living® products are not intended to diagnose, treat, cure, or prevent any disease.

NOTES:

KID'S HEALTH PROTOCOL - IMMUNITY BOOSTER SUPPORT (4 DAY PROTOCOL)

For kids 4 years and older to be taken only for 1-4 days maximum.

Supplements for this Protocol
- NingXia Red® (immunity support)
- KidScents® MightyPro™ (prebiotics and probiotics)
- Super C™ Chewables (immunity support)
- Thieves® Vitality™ (immunity support)
- Frankincense Vitality™ (immunity support)

IDEAL SUPPLEMENT SCHEDULE

Breakfast
- KidScents® MightyPro™ - Take 1 sachet.
- Super C™ Chewables - Take 1 chewable tablet.
- NingXia Red® - Drink 1-2 ounces with 1 drop Thieves® Vitality™.

Dinner
- KidScents® MightyPro™ - Take 1 sachet.
- Super C™ Chewables - Take 1 chewable tablet.
- NingXia Red® - Drink 1-2 ounces with 1-2 drops Frankincense Vitality™

How long should you use this protocol?
This protocol is meant to be used for only 1-4 days maximum. It is to rapidly support your child's immunity. Please be your child's best advocate and always check with your doctor before starting or stopping any specific regimen.

These statements have not been evaluated by the Food and Drug Administration.
Young Living® products are not intended to diagnose, treat, cure, or prevent any disease.

NOTES:

DOG HEALTH PROTOCOL - HEALTHY COAT

Supplements for this Protocol
- NingXia Red®
- Sulfurzyme™ (capsules only)
- OmegaGize3™
- Mineral Essence™

IDEAL SUPPLEMENT SCHEDULE

Breakfast
- NingXia Red® - 1 capful in their water.
- OmegaGize3™ - 1-2 capsules in their food bowl.
- Sulfurzyme™ - 1 capsule opened and sprinkled into the food bowl.
  NOTE: You may use Sulfurzyme™ powdered drink mix, but please pay close attention to their bowel movements. Too much stevia can cause diarrhea in dogs.

Dinner
- Mineral Essence™ - 1/2 dropper in food bowl.

How long should you use this protocol?
Every dog is different. Pay close attention to their behavior when introducing supplements. Please consider weight and activity level. Check with your veterinary doctor before starting or stopping any specific regimen.

These statements have not been evaluated by the Food and Drug Administration. Young Living® products are not intended to diagnose, treat, cure, or prevent any disease.

DOG HEALTH PROTOCOL - DIGESTIVE SUPPORT

Supplements for this Protocol
- NingXia Red®
- Essentialzyme™
- K & B™ Tincture
- Life 9™

IDEAL SUPPLEMENT SCHEDULE

Breakfast
- NingXia Red® - 1 capful in their water.
- Essentialzyme™ - 1/2 tablet in their food bowl.

Dinner
- K & B™ Tincture - 5 drops for small dogs or 1 dropper for large dogs in food.
- Life 9™ - 1 capsule after dinner or sprinkled in food bowl.

How long should you use this protocol?
Every dog is different. Pay close attention to their behavior when introducing supplements. Please consider weight and activity level. Check with your veterinary doctor before starting or stopping any specific regimen.

These statements have not been evaluated by the Food and Drug Administration. Young Living® products are not intended to diagnose, treat, cure, or prevent any disease.

DOG HEALTH PROTOCOL - MOBILITY SUPPORT

Depending on the size of your dog you may do this as a morning and evening regimen or only in the morning.

Supplements for this Protocol
- NingXia Red®
- AgilEase™
- Sulfurzyme™ (capsules only)

IDEAL SUPPLEMENT SCHEDULE

Breakfast
- NingXia Red® - 1 capful in their water.
- AgilEase™ - 1 capsule opened and sprinkled into the food bowl.
- Sulfurzyme™ - 1 capsule opened and sprinkled into the food bowl.
  NOTE: You may use Sulfurzyme™ powdered drink mix, but please pay close attention to their bowel movements. Too much stevia can cause diarrhea in dogs.

Dinner
- NingXia Red® - 1 capful in their water.
- AgilEase™ - 1 capsule opened and sprinkled into the food bowl.
- Sulfurzyme™ - 1 capsule opened and sprinkled into the food bowl.
  NOTE: You may use Sulfurzyme™ powdered drink mix, but please pay close attention to their bowel movements. Too much stevia can cause diarrhea in dogs.

How long should you use this protocol?
Every dog is different. Pay close attention to their behavior when introducing supplements. Please consider weight and activity level. Check with your veterinary doctor before starting or stopping any specific regimen.

These statements have not been evaluated by the Food and Drug Administration.
Young Living® products are not intended to diagnose, treat, cure, or prevent any disease.

NOTES:

CAT HEALTH PROTOCOL

There are not many supplements that a cat will readily take. Most vitamins and minerals are found in cat food. Omega-3 supplements are helpful for shedding and a shiny coat. Probiotics are helpful to keep their gut and overall immunity healthy. The following protocol is worth trying with your cat, but in the end, remember to allow your cat to choose. If they do not accept the supplements, then by all means, leave them alone and do not force them on him or her.

Supplements for this Protocol
- OmegaGize3™
- Life 9™

IDEAL SUPPLEMENT SCHEDULE

Breakfast
- OmegaGize3™ - 1 capsule in their food bowl.

Dinner
- Life 9™ - 1 capsule sprinkled in their food bowl.

How long should you use this protocol?
Every cat is different. Pay close attention to their behavior when introducing supplements. Please consider weight and activity level. Check with your veterinary doctor before starting or stopping any specific regimen.

SIDE NOTE ON ESSENTIAL OILS USE WITH CATS

Many cats (not all) lack the enzyme glucuronyl transferase which is an important liver metabolism catalyst for cytochrome P450. Without this enzyme, cats are open to potential toxicity from plants such as aloe, lilies, onions, and garlic; chocolates, pesticides, lead, zinc, caffeine, aspirin, ibuprofen, and essential oils high in phenols and terpenes. Below is a list of oils to avoid using or use highly diluted around cats.

- Phenols: Clove, Oregano, Cinnamon Bark, Tea Tree, Basil, Fennel, Oregano, Peppermint, Thyme, and Wintergreen.
- Terpenes: Tea Tree, Citrus.

The best way to approach cats with oils is to allow them to tell you what they like and don't like. They are super smart and usually come near with an oil they like or flee with an oil they don't like.

These statements have not been evaluated by the Food and Drug Administration.
Young Living® products are not intended to diagnose, treat, cure, or prevent any disease.

HORSE HEALTH

The following are supplements safe to use with your horse. Please consult with your vet prior to starting a new regimen.

Supplements to Consider
- NingXia Red™ (immunity and gut health) - 1-4 ounces per day straight, in their water, or mixed into their feed.
- Detoxzyme® (digestive enzyme) - may use up to 20 capsules per day.
- Sulfurzyme™ powder (joint support) - add 1-2 tablespoons to their feed per day.
- K&B™ Tincture (kidney and bladder support) - 10-15 drops in bottom lip gum area morning and night.
- Life 9™ (probiotic for immunity and gut health) - 2-4 capsules in their feed per day or as needed.
- DiGize™ Vitality™ (digestive support) - 10 drops in bottom lip gum area.
- Thieves® Vitality™ (immunity support) - 5 drops with equal parts carrier in bottom lip gum area.

How should I approach my horse with these supplements?
Every horse is different. Pay close attention to their behavior when introducing supplements. Check with your veterinary doctor before starting or stopping any specific regimen.

These statements have not been evaluated by the Food and Drug Administration.
Young Living® products are not intended to diagnose, treat, cure, or prevent any disease.

NOTES:

BONUS: D. GARY YOUNG'S "HAPPY" & "GREAT DAY" PROTOCOLS

Step 1: Use the "Happy" protocol every day.
This protocol was shared by D. Gary Young at a class in Wyoming in 1994.

HAPPY PROTOCOL
- Valor® - Apply on the bottoms of the feet, or a single drop on one wrist and hold the other wrist to it for a few moments to balance the entire system.
- Harmony™ - Use a single drop, over the solar plexus area (above the belly button).
- Joy™ - Apply a single drop over the heart.
- White Angelica™ - Apply a single drop in one hand, rub hands together, and brush over the head, face, chest, shoulders, down the body, right over the clothes, as though applying an angelic shield.

Step 2: Drink 1-6 ounces of NingXia Red® every day.

Step 3: Take a Longevity™ capsule every day.

Step 4: Keep Stress Away™ in your pocket and use it anytime during the day.

Step 5: Take Master Formula™ every day.

Step 6: Take 1-3 MultiGreens™ capsules once or twice a day.

Step 7: Apply Thieves® and Peppermint on the bottom of your feet every day.

Step 8: Take Sleep Essence™ before bed.

Step 9: Take Detoxzyme® before bed to help break down foods left in your system.

Step 10: Swap out all your household products for Thieves® Household Products for extra health benefits.

"Live every day in joy, gratitude, and appreciation!" ~ D. Gary Young

These statements have not been evaluated by the Food and Drug Administration.
Young Living® products are not intended to diagnose, treat, cure, or prevent any disease.

NOTES:

DISCLAIMER

The protocols and supplement descriptions in this book are based off of the usage descriptions from the Young Living® website and information readily available online. The amount and timing of each dosage are based off of the label on each product. In some instances, lower doses are recommended in this book. When you start a new supplement regimen, it is important to start slowly and pay close attention to your body. Everyone's body is unique and will respond differently. If a product does not work for you, please try another one. Check with your doctor if you are taking prescription medications. Pharmaceutical drugs should not be consumed at the same time as natural supplements. It is best to give a four hour buffer between them. Always consult your doctor when you start a new regimen.

This book gives suggestions on how to support healthy systems. It is not intended to treat or diagnose existing conditions or illnesses. Each supplement consists of multiple ingredients. Each ingredient that is listed has a basic description of what it is commonly used for in the medical and holistic practice industries. Herbs and roots have been used for centuries and the traditionally studied uses for each are readily found on sources such as PubMed, Science Direct, the National Center for Biotechnology Information, U. S. National Library of Medicine, and the Food and Drug Administration websites.

The content in this book has not been evaluated by the FDA and the supplements and protocols will not treat or cure any sickness or disease. The author is not a doctor and has published this book as a means to have a compilation of information, in one spot, to make it easier to understand the many supplements Young Living® carries.

SECTION TWO
the supplements

There are several types of supplements you will find through Young Living®. The mainstay of Young Living® is essential oils. The foundation of Young Living® is a healthy lifestyle. The founder, D. Gary Young understood how important it was to not only have the best essential oils available to consumers, but also the best, most bioavailable herbal supplements as well. It took years of commitment and research to find exactly the right sources and synergies for the supplements Young Living® carries. There are several things that set Young Living's® supplement line high above the rest: commitment to purity, commitment to research backed ingredients with proven efficacy, and the main key: infusion of essential oils into powdered herbal supplements.

For many years, the Young Living® supplement line was above average with better ingredients and better synergies of those ingredients. It was not until several years later, after many studies and tests, that Young Living® discovered infusing herbal supplements with a powdered form of essential oils made the supplements far more efficacious and bioavailable. This was a ground-breaking discovery by Gary Young that makes the Young Living® supplement line something that no other company on the planet today is able to match or even come close to. For this very reason, we will start the supplement section with the Vitality™ Line of essential oils that are specifically designed to be consumed. They are considered by the FDA as GRAS.

As stated by the FDA, "'GRAS' is an acronym for the phrase Generally Recognized As Safe. Under sections 201(s) and 409 of the Federal Food, Drug, and Cosmetic Act, any substance that is intentionally added to food is a food additive, that is subject to premarket review and approval by FDA, unless the substance is generally recognized, among qualified experts, as having been adequately shown to be safe under the conditions of its intended use, or unless the use of the substance is otherwise excepted from the definition of a food additive."

You can find a complete list of GRAS essential oils at https://tinyurl.com/GRAS-EO

VITALITY LINE ESSENTIAL OIL SUPPLEMENTS

Young Living® carries a full line of consumable essential oils, that are labeled as dietary supplements, in accordance with the FDA labeling regulations and guidelines. These oils are considered GRAS which means Generally Recognized (Regarded) as Safe for consumption. These are known essential oils used in food additives and flavorings as well as for therapeutic use. You are consuming essential oils practically every day without even knowing it. Soda pop, mints, lemon zest, orange juice, concentrated lemon juice, lemon slices in your water, spearmint gum, even eating a salad gives you essential oils.

Dr. Cole Woolley once stated that Pepsi® and Coca-Cola® use essential oils in massive amounts to flavor their products. Dr. Woolley stated, "I know the owner of a company that sells $50 million dollars of orange oil, lemon oil, tangerine oil, cinnamon oil, nutmeg oil, mandarin oil and grapefruit oil to Pepsi® and Coca-Cola® companies. He knows they go into their drinks."

This may be fascinating, but how does this help us understand the therapeutic use of these oils outside of simple flavoring agents? Let's go back to how essential oils work. Essential oils are the life-force of plants. They help the plant to regulate itself and add health and overall wellness to the cells and structure of the plant as well as act as an aroma or pheromone to attract or detract insects or invaders. These oils can work in much the same way for us as humans.

When consumed, essential oils work on our body systems. The following body systems are supported by internal use of essential oils labeled for consumption through the Vitality™ line.

- Circulatory
- Digestive and Gut
- Endocrine (hormones, sleep, energy, metabolism, etc)
- Immunity
- Lymphatic
- Nervous
- Renal and Urinary
- Respiratory

Below is each system along with the essential oils that can help support that system when used internally as a dietary supplement. Please only use essential oils from the Vitality™ line. For the best results, use an essential oil single, blend, or blend 2-3 singles from the same category to create your own blend, then add 1-2 drops of the essential oils to a capsule and top off with carrier oil such as organic olive or grapeseed oil.

Circulatory System
- Black Pepper Vitality™
- Cinnamon Bark Vitality™
- Clove Vitality™
- Dill Vitality™
- Fennel Vitality™
- Lavender Vitality™
- Lemon Vitality™
- Lemongrass Vitality™
- Marjoram Vitality™
- Nutmeg Vitality™
- Orange Vitality™
- Oregano Vitality™
- Peppermint Vitality™
- Rosemary Vitality™
- Tangerine Vitality™
- Tarragon Vitality™
- Thyme Vitality™

Digestive System
- Cardamom Vitality™ (liver, colon, digestion)
- Carrot Seed Vitality™ (liver, digestion)
- Celery seed Vitality™ (liver, digestion)
- Cinnamon Bark Vitality™ (digestion, colon)
- Coriander Vitality™ (pancreas, liver, digestion)
- DiGize™ Vitality™ blend (digestion)
- Dill Vitality™ (liver, digestion)
- Fennel Vitality™ (colon, digestion)
- GLF™ Vitality™ blend (gallbladder, liver, digestion)
- German Chamomile Vitality™ (gallbladder, liver, digestion)
- Ginger Vitality™ (digestion)
- Jade Lemon™ Vitality™ (gallbladder, liver, digestion)
- JuvaCleanse® Vitality™ blend (liver, digestion)
- JuvaFlex® Vitality™ blend (digestion)
- Lemon Vitality™ (liver, gallbladder, digestion)
- Lemongrass Vitality™ (digestion)
- Lime Vitality™ (liver, gallbladder, digestion)
- Marjoram Vitality™ (digestion)
- Nutmeg Vitality™ (liver, digestion)
- Orange Vitality™ (liver, digestion)
- Oregano Vitality™ (liver, gallbladder, colon, digestion)
- Peppermint Vitality™ (liver, gallbladder, colon, digestion)
- Rosemary Vitality™ (liver)
- Sage Vitality™ (liver)
- Spearmint Vitality™ (gallbladder, digestion)
- Tangerine Vitality™ (liver, digestion)
- Tarragon Vitality™ (colon, digestion)
- Thyme Vitality™ (colon)

Endocrine System (hormones, glands, sleep, energy, metabolism, focus, emotions)
- Black Pepper Vitality™ (energy, metabolism)
- Cinnamon Bark Vitality™ (energy, metabolism)
- Citrus Fresh™ Vitality™ blend (energy, metabolism)
- Clove Vitality™ (thyroid, energy)
- Copaiba Vitality™ (sleep, emotions, focus)
- Endoflex™ Vitality™ blend (hormones)
- Fennel Vitality™ (metabolism, hormones, PMS)
- Frankincense Vitality™ (sleep, emotions, focus)
- Grapefruit Vitality™ (energy, metabolism)
- Lavender Vitality™ (sleep, focus, emotions, hormones, PMS)
- Lemongrass Vitality™ (thyroid)
- Lime Vitality™ (metabolism, sleep, focus)
- Mountain Savory Vitality™ (energy)
- Nutmeg Vitality™ (adrenals, energy)
- Oregano Vitality™ (prostate)
- Peppermint Vitality™ (thyroid, energy, focus, emotions)
- Sage Vitality™ (prostate, hormones, metabolism, PMS)
- SclarEssence™ Vitality™ blend (hormones, PMS)
- Spearmint Vitality™ (thyroid, metabolism)
- Tangerine Vitality™ (sleep, emotions, focus)
- Tarragon Vitality™ (emotions, PMS)
- Thieves® Vitality™ blend (emotions)
- Thyme Vitality™ (prostate)

Immune System
- Basil Vitality™
- Bergamot Vitality™
- Black Pepper Vitality™
- Cinnamon Bark Vitality™
- Citrus Fresh™ Vitality™ blend
- Clove Vitality™
- Copaiba Vitality™
- Frankincense Vitality™
- GLF™ Vitality™ blend
- Ginger Vitality™
- Jade Lemon™ Vitality™
- JuvaCleanse® Vitality™ blend
- JuvaFlex® Vitality™ blend
- Laurus Nobilis Vitality™
- Lavender Vitality™
- Lemon Vitality™
- Lemongrass Vitality™
- Lime Vitality™
- Longevity™ Vitality™ blend
- Mountain Savory Vitality™
- Nutmeg Vitality™

Immune System (continued)
- Orange Vitality™
- Oregano Vitality™
- Peppermint Vitality™
- Rosemary Vitality™
- Sage Vitality™
- Spearmint Vitality™
- Tangerine Vitality™
- Thieves® Vitality™ blend
- Thyme Vitality™

Integumentary System
- Carrot Seed Vitality™ (skin)
- Clove Vitality™ (skin)
- Copaiba Vitality™ (skin, nails)
- Coriander Vitality™ (skin,
- Frankincense Vitality™ (skin, hair, nails)
- German Chamomile Vitality™ (skin)
- Jade Lemon™ Vitality™ (nails)
- Lavender Vitality™ (skin, hair, nails)
- Lemon Vitality™ (nails)
- Orange Vitality™ (skin, hair)
- Peppermint Vitality™ (hair)
- Rosemary Vitality™ (hair)

Lymphatic System
- Grapefruit Vitality™
- Jade Lemon™ Vitality™
- Lemon Vitality™
- Lemongrass Vitality™
- Lime Vitality™
- Nutmeg Vitality™
- Peppermint Vitality™
- Rosemary Vitality™
- Thieves® Vitality™ blend

Nervous System
- Cardamom Vitality™ (brain)
- Frankincense Vitality™ (brain, general)
- Lavender Vitality™ (brain, general)
- Lemongrass Vitality™ (brain)
- Orange Vitality™ (general)
- Peppermint Vitality™ (brain)
- Thyme Vitality™ (brain)

Renal/Urinary System
- Carrot Seed Vitality™ (general)
- Celery Seed Vitality™ (general)
- Citrus Fresh™ Vitality™ (general)
- Clove Vitality™ (bladder)
- Copaiba Vitality™ (kidney, bladder)
- Fennel Vitality™ (general)
- Grapefruit Vitality™ (kidney, bladder)
- Jade Lemon™ Vitality™ (kidney)
- Lavender Vitality™ (general)
- Lemon Vitality™ (kidney, bladder)
- Lemongrass Vitality™ (bladder)
- Lime Vitality™ (bladder)
- Mountain Savory Vitality™ (bladder)
- Orange Vitality™ (kidney, bladder)
- Rosemary Vitality™ (bladder)
- Tangerine Vitality™ (kidney, bladder)
- Tarragon Vitality™ (general)
- Thieves® Vitality™
- Thyme Vitality™ (bladder)

Respiratory
- Cardamom Vitality™
- Copaiba Vitality™
- Frankincense Vitality™
- Ginger Vitality™
- Laurus Nobilis Vitality™
- Lavender Vitality™
- Lemongrass Vitality™
- Lime Vitality™
- Oregano Vitality™
- Peppermint Vitality™
- Rosemary Vitality™
- Tangerine Vitality™
- Thieves® Vitality™ blend

POSSIBLE REASONS FOR NEGATIVE REACTIONS

Is your body rejecting oils or responding in unusual ways? Why do some people experience complete rejection of any and all essential oils when previously they used them without issue?

When a person overuses an essential oil internally (I can't determine if you are or not as each person is different) he or she may experience an odd reaction. This usually occurs after about two years of consuming the same thing with 20 or more drops. Sometimes the body will start to reject them in the form of rashes or what seems like an allergic response. This person may feel defeated because even simple topical or diffuser use can pose a problem.

The question I always ask when someone is having these unusual responses is, "Are you under any abnormal stress lately?" Nine times out of ten the answer is "yes". For these people, my only recommendation is to calm down and try to manage your stress. CortiStop and EndoGize are two helpful supplements.

When you are stressed out, your body creates more cortisol than normal. Your adrenals work overtime, and with larger amounts of cortisol coursing through your body, essential oils will try to help you out by attacking it. The result of their "help" is rapid and often rash-presenting detox.

Here is my advice if you find yourself having severe reactions with any and all types of essential oil use when previously there were no negative responses. I encourage you to try to manage the stress better and stop using all essential oils for 120 days to fully reset your system, and then start again. Your blood recycles fully and is brand new every 120 days. This may seem extreme but this only applies to those having major reactions. This will apply to very few people.

Please note, any full essential oil supplements need to be stopped too. Powdered supplements with powdered oils are fine. You get about the same when you eat a salad. Essential oils are present in most raw plant foods we eat, but concentrated forms of essential oil from a bottle will be too much during your reset. When you start to reintroduce essential oils again it will be like you are new, so expect two weeks of normal detox, but after that, if you are still having reactions, then I'd say stop and consider the next potential issue.

If you think it is not an overuse response then you'll need to determine several factors. Rashes happen for any number of reasons and often times people try to blame it on a topical application of some new deodorant, laundry detergent, or even natural essential oil. Topical responses to a topical application of a product is diagnosing the surface when we need to be looking at the root of the issue. It would be like wondering why a plant looks so unhealthy and trying to polish the leaves, when the soil is depleted. No amount of polishing will help the plant. Here are some questions to consider:

1. Are you under abnormal stress?
2. Have you had an unusually long period of general stress? Loss of job, loss of marriage, loss of relationship, loss of a loved one to death, moved to a new town, change in career, etc.
3. Could you possibly be going through menopause, also known as premenopause?
4. Have you started a new diet?
5. Have you started or stopped any major lifestyle habits? Exercise, hobbies, friends?
6. Could you possibly have come into contact with poison ivy or a plant protein that causes rashes?
7. Do you have an overgrowth of Candida? (Symptoms: tired all the time, thrush in your mouth, reoccurring urinary tract infections or yeast infections, sinus infections, swollen and inflamed cuticles and finger nails, joint pain, and digestive issues.)
8. Are you using essential oils and your body is on the acidic side?
9. Are you using essential oils alongside synthetic products?
10. Are you using essential oils and have not fully detoxed your body?

The last three I will go into more detail as they tend to be more in line with long-time essential oil user's issues.

ACIDIC BODY

If your body is on the acidic side (bad) rather than pH neutral (better) or slightly alkaline (best) you may experience stronger than normal detox responses. The oils will react in abnormal ways in a body that is highly acidic. You'd need to determine that on your own by checking the following areas.

Factors that contribute to acidity in the body are smoking, prescription medications, high animal protein diets, drinking alcohol or coffee, eating anything processed, eating too many processed sugars, eating too much processed wheat (bread and pasta), getting little to no exercise, not sleeping enough, plus a whole host of other things. If your body is acidic all the time, then you will experience detox responses all the time with essential oils.

The number one goal of an essential oil is to seek and destroy oxidative stress, usually in the form of acid. They want to placate it first and then give you the therapeutic action for which it is known. Essential oils will always work, but the more acidic you are, the more detox response you will have.

An interesting example of this is using lavender or other essential oils directly in your belly button. This method is highly effective for several reasons, better sleep and helping soothe stomach discomfort, but some people, when they try it, report a major rash on and around their belly button, often lasting for several days.

The belly button is a magnet for debris and build up of random toxins. Sunscreen, lotion, synthetic fibers from clothing are just a few invaders. There are thousands of bacteria found in belly buttons. The belly button is considered the "rainforest" of our body since there is such a random selection of bacteria present in each belly button.

A research team who studies belly buttons found a bacteria strain that is found only in the soil of Japan in one of their test subjects and that person had never been to Japan before. This goes to show you how international trade and possibly the clothing you buy from different countries can work like the earth's bacterial pollination playground. You can check out the whole article here: www.tinyurl.com/buttonbacteria

My recommendation is to thoroughly clean out your belly button before trying this method and use a carrier oil such as grapeseed for the first few times.

SYNTHETIC PRODUCTS
This would also translate to the personal care product a person uses. If a person decides to use essential oils, but are unwilling to give up their Bath & Body Works® soaps and lotions (honestly, it took me a while to give those up) or their favorite face or body lotion, that person will need to be prepared for the oils to potentially react badly with the synthetic fragrances, synthetic preservatives, and other synthetic ingredients that are present in most store bought products.

TOXIC BODY
The issue, however, is not only with the products we are currently using, but the toxic build-up that has been going on in our bodies for decades. We have all grown up in a world that is so vastly different than even our parents lived in. Processed synthetic greenwashing is happening all around us. Greenwashing is where a company tries to look healthy but is far from it. Our ancestral DNA does not know what to do with synthetics found in our processed foods, personal care products, household cleaning products, the plastics we type on, sit on, sleep on, and slather on, and so on and so forth; not to mention the unknown long-term damage all the electrical devices are doing to our bodies, in the form of electromagnetic radiation, that scientists have already determined to be a major cause of cancer. If your great grandparents could see us now, they would sit us all down in a corner with a great big "DUNCE" cap on.

All this to say, there could be any number of reasons someone has a negative reaction to all-natural essential oils, assuming they are, in fact, all natural, as many essential oils on the market contain synthetics as well.

The multibillion-dollar personal care industry would like us all to believe that essential oils are the problem. If we all would just use a little common sense and read the back of the labels to see what we are using, it may help clear up a lot of issues.

While this is not an exhaustive list of why you may be responding, and it may not be exactly your issues, it may be helpful information for you to help someone else down the line. Essential oils are God's gift to us, but sadly we can even mess them up too by contaminating them, overusing them or stressing ourselves out so much that they just stop working the way they are designed to work.

AGILEASE™

This delightful little gem in the supplement lineup is no joke! If you need a little (or a lot) of extra help with healthy mobility, then AgilEase™ is the one for you! This supplement is perfect if you're a gym rat, love to run or walk daily, are an athlete, or are in the middle-aged or elderly category. I'm guessing that's most of us! It supports the natural, acute inflammation response in joints after exercise. AgilEase™ helps to promote joint and cartilage health, along with more healthful mobility and flexibility through a reduction of inflammation. If you're looking for a supplement that contains Turmeric along with black pepper extract to help make the main active ingredient, curcumin, in Turmeric more bioavailable, then AgilEase™ is the best choice. Here are a few of the excellent ingredients in AgilEase™ and what they support.

INGREDIENTS
Serving Size - 2 Capsules
Servings Per Container - 30
AgilEase™ Blend - 537.5 mg
- Frankincense (Boswellia sacra) resin powder
- Calcium fructoborate (from plant minerals)
- Curcuminoids complex - Turmeric (Curcuma longa) rhizome extract
- Piperine whole fruit extract from Black Pepper (Piper nigrum)
- Collagen (with undenatured type II collagen)
- Glucosamine sulfate (not derived from shellfish).
- Hyaluronic acid (as sodium hyaluronate)
- Essential Oils - Wintergreen (Gaultheria procumbens) leaf oil, Copaiba (Copaifera officinalis) wood oil (oleoresin), Clove (Syzygium aromaticum) flower bud oil, Northern Lights Black Spruce™ (Picea mariana) whole tree oil

WHAT THE INGREDIENTS DO
- Frankincense resin powder - anti-inflammatory and anti-arthritis impacts.
- Calcium fructoborate - supports inflammation of the mucous membranes, discomfort and stiffness.
- Turmeric (curcumin longa) rhizome extract - high antioxidant and anti-inflammatory properties. Also helps increase brain function.
- Piperine extract (black pepper whole fruit) - protects liver function and helps promote the bioavailability of other supplements (helps other supplements to absorb properly).
- UC-II Undenatured collagen - protects tissue in aging joints and helps by absorbing physical impact.

WHAT THE INGREDIENTS DO (continued)

- Glucosamine sulfate - occurs naturally in the human body as fluid surrounding the joints. In supplements it is often from ground up shells from shellfish. The source used for AgilEase™ is from fermented corn.
- Hyaluronic acid - for joint pain in osteoarthritis.
- Wintergreen, Copaiba, Clove, and Northern Lights Black Spruce™ - known for their joint supporting properties.

COMMENTS FROM YOUNG LIVING

"Especially beneficial for athletes, as well as middle-aged and elderly people who may experience a natural, acute inflammation response in their joints after exercise, AgilEase™ is a joint health supplement that's perfect for healthy individuals who are looking to gain greater mobility and flexibility through the reduction of inflammation. We used unique and powerful ingredients such as frankincense powder, UC-II undenatured collagen, hyaluronic acid, calcium fructoborate, and a specially formulated proprietary essential oil blend of Wintergreen, Copaiba, Clove, and Northern Lights Black Spruce—oils that are known for their joint health benefits. Take AgilEase™ to support joint health or as a preventative measure to protect joint and cartilage health."

YOUNG LIVING STATED BENEFITS

- Supports and protects joint and cartilage health
- Beneficial for athletes and active individuals of all ages who want to support and protect their joints and cartilage
- Perfect companion to an active lifestyle, promoting healthy joint function and supporting cartilage health
- Supports the body's response to acute inflammation in healthy individuals
- Helps support healthy joint flexibility and mobility
- Formulated with ingredients and essential oils for healthy joint support
- Helps ease acute joint discomfort to improve quality of life

DIRECTIONS FOR USE

For best results, take 2 capsules daily for joint support.
You may take this anytime of the day or with a meal containing fat. While the instructions on the bottle say take anytime, and that is technically correct, the Turmeric in AgilEase™ is better absorbed when taken with fat. Piperine extract is already in this supplement so this is the best Turmeric supplement you can find.

ALKALIME® AND ALKALIME® STICK PACKS

AlkaLime® is a must for most people. It helps maintain the proper pH balance in the body. Formulated with Lemon and Lime essential oils, organic lemon powder, and biochemical mineral cell salts, this effervescent supplement formula starts working right away to soothe the occasional upset stomach. The citrus notes are sure to brighten your mood, and the mineral cell salts help support optimal pH balance in the stomach. Store a few packs in your purse or backpack and enjoy them on those hurried or stressful days when acidity soars.

INGREDIENTS
Calories - 10
Total Carbohydrate - 3 g
- Calcium (as Calcium Carbonate, Di-calcium Phosphate, Calcium Sulfate) - 201mg (15% DV)
- Sodium (as Sodium Bicarbonate, Sodium Phosphate, Sodium Sulfate) 505 mg (22% DV)
- Potassium (as Potassium Bicarbonate, Potassium Phosphate, Potassium Sulfate, Potassium Chloride) - 95mg (2% DV)

AlkaLime® Blend - 179 mg
- Lemon fruit powder
- Lemon (Citrus limon) peel oil
- Lime (Citrus aurantifolia) peel oil

Other Ingredients - Tartaric acid, Citric acid, Stevia (Stevia rebaudiana) leaf extract, Magnesium Phosphate.

WHAT THE INGREDIENTS DO
- Calcium, Sodium, Potassium - the combined negatively and positively charged biochemical mineral cell salts work in synergy to support cellular repair, nerve function, helps muscle tissues to function correctly, strengthens bones and teeth. Together they are critical to metabolic processes and they balance the biochemistry of the blood. Sodium Phosphate is an acid neutralizer.

AlkaLime® Blend -
- Lemon fruit powder, Lemon peel oil, and Lime peel oil - helps minerals absorb into the body more quickly and effectively.

Other Ingredients -
- Tartaric acid - increases the rate at which nutrients are absorbed into the bloodstream. Aids digestion by improving intestinal absorption.
- Magnesium Phosphate - Soothes stressed nerves and muscles in the body and is effective when digestive discomfort is present.

COMMENTS FROM YOUNG LIVING

"AlkaLime® is a precisely-balanced alkaline mineral complex formulated to neutralize acidity and maintain desirable pH levels in the body. Infused with Lemon and Lime essential oils and organic whole lemon powder, AlkaLime® also features enhanced effervescence and biochemical mineral cell salts for increased effectiveness. A balanced pH is thought to play an important role in maintaining overall health and vigor."

YOUNG LIVING STATED BENEFITS

- Absorbed easily and quickly by the body
- Effervescent formula starts working right away to soothe the occasional upset stomach
- Gentle on the stomach
- Helps maintain optimal pH in the stomach
- Free of artificial colors, flavors, or sweeteners, and formulated with nine biochemical mineral cell salts, the refreshing taste of Lemon and Lime essential oils, and organic lemon powder
- Comes in convenient, single-serve stick packs

DIRECTIONS FOR USE

Add 1 level teaspoon (or 1 stick pack) into 4–6 ounces of distilled or purified water. Let sit for 20–25 seconds. Gently stir until mixed, then drink immediately. Take 1–3 times daily, 1 hour before meals or bedtime as an aid in alkalizing.

The statements about the supplement and the ingredients have not been evaluated by the Food and Drug Administration. Young Living® products are not intended to diagnose, treat, cure, or prevent any disease.

NOTES:

ALLERZYME™

Allerzyme™ is the strongest of all the digestive enzymes and is the only vegan option. It is the only one containing gluten in the form of Barley grass. However some celiacs do have issues with barley grass. There is no gluten in Barley grass but there is often gluten contamination. Allerzyme™ is an excellent choice for bloating and gas and for those who are lactose intolerant. It is also good for people who like to eat desserts and items containing white processed sugar. It contains Plantain leaf, which is a natural anti-inflammatory and is packed with nutrients and vitamins. This enzyme contains the most essential oils.

INGREDIENTS
Proprietary Allerzyme™ Blend 193 mg
- Plantain (Plantago major) leaf
- Amylase
- Bromelain
- Peptidase
- Protease
- Invertase
- Phytase
- Barley (Hordeum vulgare) grass
- Lipase
- Lactase
- Cellulase
- Alpha-galactosidase
- Diastase

Proprietary Allerzyme™ Oil Blend 12 mg
- Tarragon (Artemisia dracunculus) leaf oil
- Ginger (Zingiber officinale) root oil
- Peppermint (Mentha piperita) leaf oil
- Juniper (Juniperus osteosperma) leaf oil
- Fennel (Foeniculum vulgare) seed oil
- Lemongrass (Cymbopogon flexuosus) leaf oil
- Anise (Pimpinella anisum) fruit oil
- Patchouli (Pogostemon cablin) flower oil

Other Ingredients - Hypromellose, Water, Silica.

WHAT THE INGREDIENTS DO

- Plantain leaf - digestive supporting herb.
- Amylase - breaks down starch, breads, and pasta.
- Alpha-galactosidase - breaks down polysaccharides, beans, and veggies. For gas and bloating.
- Bromelain - breaks down peptides and amino acids found in meats, dairy, eggs, and grains, as well as seeds, nuts, leafy greens, and many other foods. Works in the small intestine and supports blood to help with inflammation.
- Cellulase - breaks down man-made fiber, plant fiber, fruits, and veggies.
- Diastase (barley grass malt - gluten) - Breaks down grain sugars and starch
- Invertase - breaks down table sugar found in sweets and deserts. Breaks the connection between fructose and glucose.
- Lactase - breaks down dairy sugars. Helps with lactose intolerance.
- Lipase - breaks down dietary fats and oils. Helps liver function.
- Peptidase - finishes breaking down Proteases. Helps support the immune system and inflammation.
- Phytase - helps with bone health and pulls needed minerals from grains making them bioavailable.
- Protease 3.0 - supports blood circulation and toxicity. Higher acid content to break down animal protein.
- Protease 4.5 - helps with sinusitis and has a lower acidic content.
- Protease 6.0 - helps with edema and carries away toxins. Helps reduce pain and varicose veins. Works in the blood. Least acidic.
- Barley (Hordeum vulgare) grass - supports digestion and helps reduce constipation.
- Tarragon, Ginger, Peppermint, Juniper, Fennel, Lemongrass, Anise, and Patchouli - supports digestion and bioavailability.

COMMENTS FROM YOUNG LIVING

"Allerzyme™ is a vegetarian enzyme complex that promotes digestion. For the relief of occasional symptoms such as fullness, pressure, bloating, gas, pain, and/or minor cramping that may occur after eating."

DIRECTIONS FOR USE

Take 1 capsule three times daily just prior to all meals or as needed. Indications - For the relief of occasional symptoms such as fullness, pressure, bloating, gas, pain, and/or minor cramping that may occur after eating.

Warning - Do not give to children under 12 years of age except under the supervision of a doctor. If symptoms persist, discontinue use of this product and consult your physician. Keep in a cool dry place. Do not expose to excessive heat or direct sunlight. If pregnant or under a doctor's care, consult your physician.

The statements about the supplement and the ingredients have not been evaluated by the Food and Drug Administration. Young Living® products are not intended to diagnose, treat, cure, or prevent any disease.

AMINOWISE™

AminoWise™ is one of those special necessities for those of us who love to get in a good hard workout or also for those who need extra amino acids to help with your circulatory system. You can drink this during your workout or directly after to help your body flush lactic acid buildup. Your body will be so happy you added this to your workout! I promise, your cells will smile!

INGREDIENTS
Calories 10
Total Carbohydrates 5 g
- Vitamin E (as d-alpha-tocopherol acetate) 10.8 mg (70% DV)
- Calcium (as calcium citrate) 3 mg (<1%)
- Magnesium (as manesium citrate) 2 mg (<1%)
- Zinc (as zinc gluconate) 1.4 mg (10%)
- Sodium (as sodium citrate) 46 mg (2%)
- Potassium (as potassium citrate) 12 mg (<1%)

AminoWise™ Muscle Performance Blend 5.7 g
Branched-chain amino acids (2:1:1 leucine, iso-leucine, valine), L-citrulline, L-glutamine, B-alanine, L-arginine, L-taurine
AminoWise™ Recovery Blend 1.2 g
NingXia wolfberry (Lycium barbarum) fruit powder, Lime (Citrus latifolia) fruit powder, Polyphenols extract, Zinc, Vitamin E, Lemon (Citrus limon) peel oil, Lime (Citrus latifolia) rind oil
AminoWise™ Hydration Mineral Blend 277 mg
Sodium citrate, Potassium citrate, Calcium citrate, Magnesium citrate

Other Ingredients - Fructo-oligosaccharides, Tapioca maltodextrin, Citric acid, Natural flavors, Calcium silicate, Stevia (Stevia rebaudiana) leaf extract, Silica, and Tapioca starch.

WHAT THE INGREDIENTS DO
- Vitamin E - supports immune function, prevents inflammation, promotes eye health.
- Calcium citrate - supports bone loss.
- Magnesium citrate - supports the normal functioning of cells, nerves, muscles, bones, and heart.
- Zinc - promotes a healthy immune system. Aids in healing of wounds.
- Sodium citrate - helps to alkalinize the urine.
- Potassium citrate - helps to decrease the risk of stroke, lower blood pressure, protect against loss of muscle mass, preserve bone mineral density, and reduce kidney stones.
- Branched-chain amino acids (2-1-1 leucine, iso-leucine, valine) - promotes healthy pathways to support weakness, supports signs of loss of brain function due to severe liver damage, reduces fatigue during exercise, promote wound healing, and stimulates insulin production.
- Polyphenols extract - helps digestion, helps protect tissue against oxidative stresses.
- NingXia wolfberry fruit powder - Natural polysaccharide that supports the healthy function of the immune system, as well as healthy regeneration of tissues and cells.

Amino Acids
- L-citrulline - helps open veins and arteries to increase blood flow and reduce blood pressure.
- L-glutamine - boosts immune cell activity in the gut, helps prevent infection and inflammation.
- B-alanine - improves athletic function and exercise capacity, aids in building lean muscle mass.
- L-arginine - stimulates the release of growth hormones and insulin, promotes increased blood flow.
- L-taurine - promotes cardiovascular health, lowers risk of disease, increases sports performance.

Citrus Powder and Oils
- Lime fruit powder - promotes weight loss, improves skin quality, improves immune system, promotes consumption of water.
- Lemon peel oil - natural detoxifier, promotes weight loss, boosts immune system and energy.
- Lime peel oil - boosts immune system, natural detoxifier.

COMMENTS FROM YOUNG LIVING

"Optimize your workout recovery with the triple-targeted formula of AminoWise™. It uses three blends for one powerful result - The Muscle Performance blend aids muscle building and repair, the Recovery blend helps reduce muscle fatigue, and the Hydration Mineral blend replenishes important minerals lost during exercise. Simply mix 1 scoop with water and drink immediately after your workout to ensure that you're getting the most out of your hard work. AminoWise™ was developed and formulated to fill a need within the nutritional product line as a during and after-workout replenishing boost for the muscles. With a hydrating blend of minerals that are lost during exercise and with no added sugars, artificial sweeteners, preservatives, or artificial colors or flavors, AminoWise™ is a standout in the field of workout supplementation."

DIRECTIONS FOR USE

Mix 1 scoop with 8 fl. oz. of water and consume during or after exercise.

The statements about the supplement and the ingredients have not been evaluated by the Food and Drug Administration. Young Living® products are not intended to diagnose, treat, cure, or prevent any disease.

BALANCE COMPLETE™

Balance Complete™ is the perfect meal replacement shake mix that will keep you going until your next meal. With 11 grams of protein and 170 calories, this shake packs a punch with fiber, vitamins, and minerals. Add a drop of Tangerine Vitality™ and Cinnamon Bark Vitality™ for an extra kick!

INGREDIENTS
Calories - 170
Total Fat - 6 g (9% DV)
Cholesterol - 30 mg (10% DV)
Sodium - 115 mg (5% DV)
Potassium - 330 mg (9% DV)
Carbohydrate - 26 g (9% DV)
Protein - 11g

- A - (25% DV)
- C (ascorbic acid) - (25% DV)
- D3 (Cholecalciferol) - (25% DV)
- E - (15% DV)
- B1 (Thiamine HCI) - (25% DV)
- B2 (Riboflavin) - (25% DV)
- B3 (Niacin) - (30% DV)
- B6 (Pyridoxine HCI) - (25% DV)
- Folate - (30% DV)
- B12 (Methylcobalamin) - (35% DV)
- B7 (Biotin) - (30% DV)
- Calcium - (40% DV)
- Iron - (2% DV)
- Pantothenic Acid - (25% DV)
- Phosphorus - (25% DV)
- Iodine (Potassium iodide) - (25% DV)
- Magnesium - (35% DV)
- Zinc - (25% DV)
- Selenium - (30% DV)
- Chromium - (30% DV)
- Molybdenum - (20% DV)
- Whey protein concentrate
- Natural flavors
- Nonfat dry milk
- MCT (Medium-chain triglycerides)
- Fructose
- Lecithin
- Calcium (Tricalcium phosphate)

Proprietary V-Fiber™ Blend
- Larch polysaccharides, NingXia wolfberry (Lycium barbarum) fruit, Brown rice bran, Guar gum, Konjac, Xanthan gum, Chicory root (Cichorium intybus) fiber extract (FOS), Sodium alginate

Proprietary Enzyme Complex
- Lactase, Lipase, Bromelain, Papain, Amylase

Additional Ingredients
- Xylitol, Magnesium oxide, Barley (Hordeum vulgare) grass, Neohesperidin derivate (flavor from natural citrus), Cinnamon (Cinnamomum verum) bark, Mixed carotenoids (Vitamin A), Lo han kuo fruit extract, Barley grass (Hordeum vulgare) juice, Aloe vera leaf, Beta-carotene, B5 (Pantothenic acid from calcium pantothenate), B6 (Pyridoxine HCI), Chromium amino nicotinate, B9 Folic acid, Orange (Citrus sinensis) peel oil

WHAT THE INGREDIENTS DO
Proprietary V-Fiber™ Blend
- Larch polysaccharides - source of dietary fiber potent in biological immune-enhancing properties which promote healthy regeneration of tissues and cells.
- NingXia wolfberry (Lycium barbarum) fruit - natural polysaccharide that supports the healthy function of the immune system, as well as healthy regeneration of tissues and cells.
- Brown rice bran - natural source of dietary fiber that promotes proper digestive function. It is nutrient-rich in bioavailable vitamins, minerals and antioxidants.
- Guar gum - stabilizes ingredients to keep fats and oils from separating. Helps promote regular bowel movements by holding water in the intestines which help form healthy stool.
- Konjac - natural source of fiber known to be low in calories and very high in fiber. Promotes a feeling of fullness along with motivating bowel movements which encourages colon health.
- Xanthan gum - natural emulsifier that promotes healthy stool; positively affects expediting digestion.
- Chicory root (Cichorium intybus) fiber extract (FOS) - soluble plant fiber that boosts digestion, curbs appetite, naturally supports cardiovascular health and improves bowel and gut health. Considered a type of prebiotic.
- Sodium alginate - brown algae source of sodium salt used as an emulsifier.

Proprietary Enzyme Complex - Digestive enzymes
- Lactase - breaks down dairy sugars. Helps with lactose intolerance.
- Lipase - breaks down dietary fats and oils. Helps liver function.
- Bromelain - breaks down peptides and amino acids found in foods. Works in the small intestine and supports blood to help with inflammation.
- Papain - digestive aid, and may help with parasites, psoriasis, shingles, diarrhea, runny nose, plus others.
- Amylase - breaks down starch, breads, and pasta.

Vitamins and Minerals
- Vitamin A - phytonutrients that support cellular communication and fight free radicals.
- Vitamin C (ascorbic acid) - slows the effects of aging by protecting against free radical damage and oxidative stress, supports the immune system, counteracts the negative effects of sun damage, cigarette smoke, air pollution and other environmental stressors, which promote healthy cardiovascular functioning. Supports the body's natural ability to form collagen which maintains healthy connective tissue, including the skin, bones, joints and blood vessels. Supports eye health and helps with absorption of iron.
- Vitamin B (Niacinamide) - a form of Vitamin B6 which is important to support the maintenance health of nerves, skin, and red blood cells.
- Calcium (Tricalcium phosphate) - helps prevent bone loss.
- Magnesium oxide - supports immunity, nerves, heart, eyes, brain and muscles.

- Zinc oxide - trace mineral that supports immunity and blood health.
- Mixed tocopherols (Vitamin E) - fat soluble. High antioxidant property.
- Selenium (Selenomethionine) - supports normal cardiovascular function as a powerful antioxidant that defends against free radicals in the body.
- Beta-carotene - acts as an antioxidant, protects cells from free radical damage.
- Molybdenum citrate - trace mineral that is an essential nutrient that acts as a cofactor for essential enzymes which drive important chemical reactions in the body to convert, break down and remove toxic by products of metabolism.
- Vitamin B5 (Pantothenic acid from calcium pantothenate) - promotes healthy skin, supports the nervous system, proper digestion, creates red blood cells that carry oxygen to our cells, and is essential to hormone production within the adrenal glands.
- Vitamin B6 (Pyridoxine HCl) - supports the maintenance health of nerves, skin, and red blood cells.
- Chromium amino nicotinate - boosts metabolism and promotes improvement in blood sugar control in the body.
- Vitamin B1 (Thiamine HCl) - supports a healthy nervous system and promotes healthy cardiovascular function by breaking down fats and proteins. Functions by converting carbohydrates into glucose to improve energy and helps the body withstand stress while maintaining a healthy metabolism.
- Vitamin B2 (Riboflavin) - needed for overall growth. It also helps support energy levels.
- Vitamin D3 - supports bones and immunity. Helps boost weight loss, and improves moods.
- Vitamin B12 (Methylcobalamin) - the most bioavailable form of B12. Plays an important role in red blood cell production. Supports brain health, eye health, skin health, DNA production, cardiovascular health, and converts food into energy.
- Biotin (B7) - helps the body convert food into energy.
- Folic acid (as folate) - required by FDA to be listed as folic acid (synthesized version); folic acid derived from natural sources is folate. Folate is needed for your body to make DNA. Having enough folate may prevent iron deficiency. It helps promote hair, skin and nail health through cell regeneration. Folate is an important supplement for pregnant women by helping prevent certain birth defects. It is also noted that folate supports your mood by transforming amino acids from your food into neurotransmitters such as serotonin and dopamine.
- Iodine (Potassium iodide) - a trace mineral that is an essential component of the thyroid hormones; it controls metabolic rate, maintains healthy energy levels, facilitates the removal of toxins in the body, boosts immunity and is critical in the prevention of enlarged thyroid gland.

Other Ingredients
- Whey protein concentrate - high in amino acids; stimulates muscle growth.
- MCT (Medium-chain triglycerides) - supports cardiovascular health.
- Natural flavors - improve taste.
- Nonfat dry milk - protein source.
- Fructose - fruit or honey sugar.
- Lecithin - rich in choline - beneficial to brain health.
- Xylitol - naturally occurring plant-based sugar alcohol. 40% fewer calories than sugar.
- Barley (Hordeum vulgare) grass - supports digestion and helps reduce constipation.
- Barley grass (Hordeum vulgare) juice - promotes improved digestive function.
- Aloe vera leaf - rich in antioxidant properties; it soothes and aides in digestion.
- Neohesperidin derivate (flavor from natural citrus) - citrus based sweetener.
- Lo han kuo fruit extract - monk fruit adds sweetness with no calories.
- Cinnamon (Cinnamomum verum) bark - supports blood glucose and adds flavor.
- Orange peel oil - enhances immunity, improves blood flow and assists a healthy blood pressure; can be calming and uplifting; helps reduce signs of aging in skin and promotes the production of collagen; beneficial for oral health.

COMMENTS FROM YOUNG LIVING
"Balance Complete™ is a super-food-based meal replacement that is both a powerful nutritive energizer and a cleanser. Offering the benefits of NingXia wolfberry powder, brown rice bran, barley grass, extra virgin coconut oil, aloe vera, cinnamon powder, and our premium whey protein blend, Balance Complete™ is high in fiber, high in protein, and contains the good fats, enzymes, vitamins, and minerals needed for a nutritionally dynamic meal. Balance Complete™ also features Young Living's proprietary V-Fiber™ blend, which supplies an amazing 11 grams of fiber per serving, absorbs toxins, and satisfies the appetite while balancing the body's essential requirements."

DIRECTIONS FOR USE
Add 2 scoops of Balance Complete™ to 8-10 ounces of cold water or the milk of your choice. Shake, stir or blend until smooth. For added flavor, add fruit or essential oils. During Young Living's five-day nutritive cleanse, replace your three daily meals with Balance Complete™ and follow recommended schedule. For daily health maintenance, replace your least nutritious meal with Balance Complete™. For weight management programs, replace two daily meals with Balance Complete™.

The statements about the supplement and the ingredients have not been evaluated by the Food and Drug Administration. Young Living® products are not intended to diagnose, treat, cure, or prevent any disease.

BLM™

BLM™ stands for bones, ligaments, and muscles. BLM™ is an excellent addition to your mobility support regimen. It helps improve flexibility and reduces inflammation while boosting immune function. Infused with essential oils known to help support circulation and soothe muscles, this supplement may be combined with AgilEase™ and/or Sulfurzyme™ or taken by itself.

INGREDIENTS
- Glucosamine Sulfate (derived from shellfish)
- Collagen type II (chicken sternum extract)
- MSM (methylsulfonylmethane)
- Balsam Canada (Abies Balsamea) leaf/branch oil
- Wintergreen (Gaultheria procumbens) leaf oil
- Manganese (as manganese citrate)
- Clove (Syzygium aromaticum) flower bud oil

Other Ingredients - Rice Flour, Gelatin, Magnesium stearate, Silicone dioxide

WHAT THE INGREDIENTS DO
- Glucosamine Sulfate - produces chemicals involved in building tendons, ligaments, cartilage and synovial fluid (the thick fluid that surrounds joints). (derived from shellfish).
- Collagen type II (chicken sternum extract) - may improve joint flexibility, comfort and physical functions; supports gut integrity that helps boost the immune system; helps form elastin and other compounds to help maintain skin's youthful appearance; supports healthy digestive function.
- MSM - decreases joint and muscle discomfort, significantly reduces inflammation in the body, and inhibits the breakdown of cartilage.
- Balsam Canada (Abies Balsamea) leaf/branch oil - soothes muscle discomfort and supports respiratory function.
- Wintergreen - useful to relieve discomfort and stimulate relaxation.
- Manganese - supports bone health, antioxidant activity, healthy blood sugar level management, and metabolic support.
- Clove oil - improves circulation, reduces inflammation, and boosts immunity.

COMMENTS FROM YOUNG LIVING
"BLM™ supports normal bone and joint health. This formula combines powerful natural ingredients, such as type II collagen, MSM, glucosamine sulfate, and manganese citrate, enhanced with therapeutic-grade essential oils. These ingredients have been shown to support healthy cell function and encourage joint health and fluid movement."

DIRECTIONS FOR USE
If you weigh less than 120 lbs., take 1 capsule 3 times daily. If you weigh between 120 and 200 lbs., take 1 capsule 4 times daily. If you weigh over 200 lbs., take 1 capsule 5 times daily. Allow 4-8 weeks of daily use before expecting noticeable results.

NOTE: Keep in a cool dry place. Keep out of the reach of children. Do not expose to excessive heat or direct sunlight. If pregnant or under a doctor's care, consult your physician.

The statements about the supplement and the ingredients have not been evaluated by the Food and Drug Administration. Young Living® products are not intended to diagnose, treat, cure, or prevent any disease.

CARDIOGIZE™

CardioGize™ was one of D. Gary Young's (Young Living's founder) last formulations. The cardiovascular system is one of the most important systems in the body as it directly affects every other system. CardioGize™ is an excellent choice for all adults and will help boost antioxidant support as well as keep you moving in the right direction.

INGREDIENTS
Carbohydrates 1 g
- Vitamin K (as K2 menaquinone-7) 100 mcg (80% DV)
- Folate (from Lemon peel extract) 165 mcg DFE (41% DV)
- Selenium (from yeast) 100 mcg (180% DV)

Proprietary Healthy Heart Blend 1255 mg
- Garlic bulb extract [deodorized]
- CoQ10 [90-100 mg/serving]
- Astragalus root powder
- Dong Quai root powder
- Motherwort herb powder
- Cat's claw bark powder
- Hawthorn berry powder
- Cactus cladode powder
- Cardamom seed powder

Proprietary CardioGize™ Essential Oil Blend 25 mg
- Angelica, Cardamom, Cypress, Lavender, Helichrysum, Rosemary, Cinnamon

Other ingredients - Hypromellose, Water, Silica

WHAT THE INGREDIENTS DO
- K2 - helps push calcium into bones preventing buildup in the coronary blood vessels.
- Folate - plant-based source of Vitamin B9. Helps cells divide.
- Selenium - supports normal cardiovascular function. Works synergistically with CoQ10.
- Garlic bulb extract - supports healthy circulation.
- CoQ10 - helps the body produce energy, normal growth, maintenance and repair.
- Astragalus root powder - supports immunity.
- Dong Quai root powder - nourishing to female glands, good for circulation.
- Motherwort herb powder - cardiovascular support. Helps to ease nervous tension.
- Cat's claw bark powder - helps the blood to flow smoother and healthier.
- Hawthorn berry powder - improves blood flow and protects blood vessels.
- Cactus cladode powder - high in beneficial fibers and antioxidants.
- Cardamom seed powder - rich in antioxidant benefits, influences healthy cholesterol levels, circulation and blood flow to protect cardiovascular health.

COMMENTS FROM YOUNG LIVING
Formulated by D. Gary Young, CardioGize™ supports healthy heart function and blood circulation and may promote a higher quality of life. This supplement uses the proper synergistic ratio of CoQ10 and selenium, while garlic and CoQ10 provide antioxidant properties and vitamin K2 supports healthy vascular system function."

DIRECTIONS FOR USE
Recommended 2 capsules daily for children and adults over the age of 12 with food.
NOTE: Keep out of the reach of children. If you are pregnant, nursing, taking medication, or have a medical condition, consult a health professional prior to use. Not recommended while using blood thinners. Please check with personal physician if taking medication contraindicated before using CardioGize™.

The statements about the supplement and the ingredients have not been evaluated by the Food and Drug Administration. Young Living® products are not intended to diagnose, treat, cure, or prevent any disease.

COMFORTONE™

ComforTone® is the perfect supplement to support your stomach, digestion, liver, and gallbladder. It has herbs and roots to help with the elimination process. It is also known to help soothe discomfort from foods and will help to placate gas.

INGREDIENTS
ComforTone® Blend – 694mg
- Cascara Sagrada bark
- Psyllium seed
- Barberry bark
- Burdock root
- Fennel seed
- Garlic bulb
- Echinacea root
- Bentonite
- Diatomaceous earth
- Ginger root
- German Chamomile flower extract
- Apple pectin
- Licorice root
- Cayenne fruit

ComforTone® Essential Oils
Tarragon, Ginger, Tangerine, Rosemary, Anise, Peppermint, Ocotea, German Chamomile
Other ingredients - Gelatin, Water, Silicon dioxide

WHAT THE INGREDIENTS DO
- Cascara Sagrada bark - helps to support normal intestinal peristalsis (wave-like motion that moves waste out of the body). NOTE - Turns stool black and is a laxative.
- Psyllium seed - helps speed the passage of stool through the digestive tract.
- Barberry bark - helps remove morbid matter from the stomach and bowels.
- Burdock root - supports the kidneys and lymphatic system.
- Fennel seed - improves digestion, helps digestion, and is an appetite suppressant.
- Garlic bulb - stimulates the lymphatic system to help throw off waste.
- Echinacea root - supports immunity, digestion, and lymphatic filtration.
- Bentonite - protects intestinal lining, neutralizes bacteria in the gut.
- Diatomaceous earth - soft fibers that absorb toxins to be eliminated.
- Ginger root - calms and cleanses bowels, minimizes flatulence.
- German Chamomile flower extract - helps upset stomach and gas.
- Apple pectin - natural source of dietary fiber.
- Licorice root - mild laxative. Softens, lubricates and nourishes the intestinal tract.
- Cayenne fruit - rebuilds tissue in the stomach and supports digestion.

ComforTone™ Essential Oils
- Tarragon, Ginger, Tangerine, Rosemary, Anise, Peppermint, Ocotea, German Chamomile - supports proper digestion.

COMMENTS FROM YOUNG LIVING
"ComforTone® (capsules) is an effective combination of herbs and essential oils that support the health of the digestive system by eliminating residues from the colon and enhancing its natural ability to function optimally. Because it supports normal peristalsis (the wave-like contractions that move food through the intestines), ComforTone® is ideal for strengthening the system that delivers nutrients to the rest of the body. It also contains ingredients that are beneficial to liver, gallbladder, and stomach health."

DIRECTIONS FOR USE
Take 1 capsule 3 times daily. Drink at least 64 ounces of distilled water throughout the day for best results.

The statements about the supplement and the ingredients have not been evaluated by the Food and Drug Administration. Young Living® products are not intended to diagnose, treat, cure, or prevent any disease.

CORTISTOP®

CortiStop® is a favorite of those who need a little help with the jitters. When life is coming at you from all sides, this is what to take first thing in the morning. Men can use it too, even though Young Living® mentions it is for women. Cortistop® contains powerful precursor hormones pregnenolone and DHEA derived from wild yams. It supports emotional fluctuations and helps improve memory and cognitive function. Cortistop® is an excellent choice to support women who experience PMS or are going through menopause. It is designed to help control and regulate healthy cortisol production during times of additional stress. See each ingredient below along with the benefits of each.

INGREDIENTS
- Pregnenolone
- L-a-phosphatidylserine
- L-a-phosphatidylcholine
- Black cohosh (Actaea racemosa) root extract
- DHEA [derived from wild yam (Dioscorea Villosa) Root]
- Clary Sage (Salvia sclarea) flowering top
- Conyza canadensis flowering top
- Fennel (Foeniculum vulgare) seed
- Frankincense (Boswellia carteri) gum/resin
- Peppermint (Mentha piperita) leaf

WHAT THE INGREDIENTS DO
- Pregnenolone - precursor hormone that increases the production of all hormones in the body such as progesterone, estrogen, and cortisol. It combats fatigue, increases energy, supports memory, supports motivation, helps increase libido, and may help improve mood swings.
- L-a-phosphatidylserine - improves mental function.
- L-a-phosphatidylcholine - improves memory function and memory loss.
- Black cohosh root - supports menopause and PMS.
- DHEA dehydroepiandrosterone - precursor hormone that helps with cognition, emotions, libido, and muscle and bone mass. May help with vaginal dryness.
- Clary Sage, Canadian Fleabane, Fennel, Frankincense, and Peppermint - all hormone supporting essential oils.

COMMENTS FROM YOUNG LIVING
CortiStop® is a proprietary dietary supplement designed to help the body maintain its natural balance and harmony. When under stress, the body produces cortisol. When cortisol is produced too frequently, it can have negative health consequences such as feelings of fatigue, difficulty maintaining healthy weight, and difficulty maintaining optimal health of cardiovascular systems. CortiStop supports the glandular systems of women.

DIRECTIONS FOR USE
Take 2 capsules in the morning before breakfast. If desired, for extra benefits, take another 2 capsules before retiring. Use daily for eight weeks. Discontinue use for 2-4 weeks before once more resuming.

The statements about the supplement and the ingredients have not been evaluated by the Food and Drug Administration. Young Living® products are not intended to diagnose, treat, cure, or prevent any disease.

DETOXZYME®

Detoxzyme® is an enzyme powerhouse to help you cleanse your system. It is an excellent choice for bloating and gas, and for those who are lactose intolerant. Detoxzyme® helps to flush the body of dead white blood cells to allow you to function at your best. Cumin powder is added to Detoxzyme® and provides natural iron and also helps with blood sugar. It is also a good choice if you have a sweet tooth. It contains the fewest essential oils of the adult enzymes and is not Vegan. Below is a list of the enzymes in Detoxzyme® and their function.

INGREDIENTS

- Amylase
- Cumin (Cminum cyminum) seed powder
- Invertase
- Protease 4.5
- Glucoamylase
- Bromelain
- Phytase
- Lipase
- Cellulase
- Alpha-galactosidase
- Lactase

Essential Oils - Cumin (Cuminum cyminum) seed oil, Anise (Pimpinella anisum) seed oil, Fennel (Foeniculum vulgare) seed oil
Other ingredients - Hypromellose, Rice Bran, Silica, Magnesium Stearate, Water

WHAT THE INGREDIENTS DO

- Alpha-galactosidase - breaks down beans, and veggies (for gas and bloating).
- Amylase - breaks down starches, breads, and pasta.
- Bromelain - breaks down meats, dairy, eggs, and grains, as well as seeds, nuts, leafy greens, and other foods. Supports blood to help with inflammation.
- Cellulase - breaks down man-made fiber, plant fiber, fruits, and veggies.
- Glucoamylase - breaks down starch and cereals. Flushes dead white blood cells.
- Invertase - breaks down table sugar found in sweets and deserts. Breaks the connection between fructose and glucose.
- Lactase - breaks down dairy sugars. Helps with lactose intolerance.
- Lipase - breaks down dietary fats and oils. Helps liver function.
- Phytase - helps with bone health and pulls needed minerals from grains.
- Protease 4.5 - helps with sinusitis and has a lower acidic content.
- Digestive Supporting Herb - Cumin
- Digestive Supporting Essential Oils - Cumin, Anise, Fennel

COMMENTS FROM YOUNG LIVING

"Detoxzyme® combines a myriad of powerful enzymes that complete digestion, help detoxify, and promote cleansing. The ingredients in Detoxzyme® also work with the body to support normal function of the digestive system, which is essential for maintaining and building health."

DIRECTIONS FOR USE

Take 2 capsules 3 times daily between meals or as needed. This product may be used in conjunction with a cleansing or detoxifying program. For the relief of occasional symptoms such as fullness, pressure, bloating, gas, pain, and/or minor cramping that may occur after eating.

The statements about the supplement and the ingredients have not been evaluated by the Food and Drug Administration. Young Living® products are not intended to diagnose, treat, cure, or prevent any disease.

DIGEST & CLEANSE™

Digest & Cleanse™ is oh so helpful for those of us who have tummy troubles. It can become your best friend! I highly recommend having this in your stash and taking it on a regular basis.

INGREDIENTS

Digest & Cleanse™ Blend 710mg
Contains 12 drops total of Coconut carrier and pure essential oils.
- Medium chain triglycerides (from fractionated Coconut oil)
- Peppermint (Montha piperita) aerial parts oil
- Caraway (Carum carvi) fruit oil
- Coconut (Cocus nucifera) fruit oil
- Lemon (Citrus limon) peel oil
- Ginger (Zingiber officinale) root oil
- Fennel (Foeniculum vulgare) seed oil
- Anise (Pimpinella anisum) seed oil

Other Ingredients - Hypromellose, Water, Silica
Contains tree nuts (Coconut)

WHAT THE INGREDIENTS DO
- Medium chain triglycerides - may help burn fat and reduce hunger.
- Peppermint oil - increases energy and improves digestion.
- Caraway oil - antioxidant that promotes digestion and increases weight loss.
- Coconut oil - enhances the immune system, protects the liver from toxins, reduces inflammation, improves digestion, helps burn fat, reduces hunger.
- Lemon oil - improves digestion and stimulates lymphatic drainage.
- Ginger oil - improves digestion, reduces inflammation, and supports the liver.
- Fennel oil - improves digestion, supports blood pressure, supports weight loss.
- Anise oil - helps keep blood sugar levels stable, improves digestion.

COMMENTS FROM YOUNG LIVING
"Digest & Cleanse™ soothes gastrointestinal upset and supports healthy digestion. Stress, overeating, and toxins can irritate the gastrointestinal system and cause cramps, gas, and nausea that interfere with the body's natural digestive and detox functions. Supplementing with Digest & Cleanse™ will soothe the bowel, prevent gas, and stimulate stomach secretions, thus aiding digestion. Digest & Cleanse™ is formulated with clinically proven and time-tested essential oils that work synergistically to help prevent occasional indigestion and abdominal pain. Precision Delivery softgels release in the intestines for optimal absorption and targeted relief and to help prevent aftertaste. This product can also be used in conjunction with any cleansing program, such as Young Living's 5-Day Nutritive Cleanse. Digest & Cleanse™ is part of the new Purely Oils line of premium essential oil supplements."

DIRECTIONS FOR USE
Take 1 softgel 1 to 3 times daily with water 30-60 minutes prior to meals.
Caution - Keep out of the reach of children.
If pregnant or if you have a medical condition, consult with a healthcare professional before use.

The statements about the supplement and the ingredients have not been evaluated by the Food and Drug Administration. Young Living® products are not intended to diagnose, treat, cure, or prevent any disease.

ENDOGIZE™

EndoGize™ is a strong endocrine supporting supplement for both men and women. It contains Ashwagandha root powder which is one of the most important herbs used in Ayurvedic medicine, an ancient practice that began in India 3,000 years ago and is still in use today. The root comes from India, Africa, and the Middle East and has a common name of Indian ginseng because of its energizing properties, but it is not ginseng. The plant is more like a tomato plant. "Ashwa" means horse. Ashwagandha gets its name because it smells like a horse.

Ashwagandha root has been touted to help adrenal fatigue, support inflammation in the body, boost testosterone levels, help increase fertility in men, help to lower blood sugar levels, improve insulin sensitivity in muscle cells, improve memory and brain function, help reduce cortisol levels when chronically stressed, and also support healthy emotions, peace, and stress.

Other herbs and phytonutrients in EndoGize™ are used for libido support and the overall health of the endocrine system. It contains natural DHEA found in wild yams, which is helpful for mood swings, night sweats, and general hormone support for both women and men.

There are several digestive enzymes in EndoGize™ making this supplement helpful to stressed individuals. High levels of chronic stress can cause digestive enzyme production to decrease. Using EndoGize™ will help support healthy digestion while rebuilding the strength of your endocrine system.

INGREDIENTS
- Ashwagandha (Withania somnifera) root powder
- Muira puama (Ptychopetalum olacoides) bark
- L-arginine
- Epimedium (Epimedium sagittatum) aerial parts
- Tibulus (Tribulus terrestris) fruit extract
- Phosphatidylcholine
- Lecithin (Soy)
- DHEA (dehydroepiandrosterone)
- Black pepper (Piper nigrum) fruit extract
- Glucoamylase, Acid stable protease
- Longjack (Eurycoma longifolia) root extract
- Amylase
- Cellulase

EndoGize™ Oil Blend 34 mg
- Ginger (Zingiber officinale) root oil
- Myrrh (commiphora myrrha) gum/resin oil
- Cassia (Cinnamomum aromaticum) Branch/leaf oil
- Clary sage (Saliva sclarea) flowering tip oil
- Canadian fleabane (Conyza canadensis) flowering top

WHAT THE INGREDIENTS DO

- Ashwagandha root powder - supports immunity, mental clarity, concentration, and alertness. May help boost testosterone levels, may help increase fertility in men, may help to lower blood sugar levels, may improve insulin sensitivity in muscle cells, may improve memory and brain function, may help reduce cortisol levels when chronically stressed, and may support healthy emotions, peace, and stress.
- Muira puama bark - helps improve libido and Erectile Dysfunction.
- L-arginine - an amino acid that helps support the circulatory system allowing improved blood flow.
- Epimedium aerial parts (aka "Horny Goat Weed") - used to support Erectile Dysfunction and sexual drive.
- Tribulus fruit extract - supports a healthy urinary tract, helps improve libido, and possibly increase testosterone. Supports body building.
- Phosphatidylcholine - some research suggests it may improve symptoms of ulcerative colitis. It helps with memory and also may help break down fat.
- Soy Lecithin - a fat that helps with memory. It may also help support healthy emotions, peace, eczema, the gallbladder and liver.
- DHEA dehydroepiandrosterone (from wild yams) - precursor hormone that helps with cognition, healthy emotions, libido, and muscle and bone mass. It may also help with vaginal dryness.
- Black pepper fruit extract - improves digestion, helps metabolism, promotes energy, supports inflammation response, and helps other supplements become more bioavailable.
- Longjack root extract - supports energy, sexual desire, and male fertility.

Digestive Enzymes

- Glucoamylase - breaks down starchy foods and cereals. Flushes the body of dead white blood cells.
- Protease 6.0 - helps with edema and carries away toxins. Helps reduce pain and varicose veins. Works in the blood. Least acidic.
- Cellulase - breaks down man-made fiber, plant fiber, fruits, and veggies.
- Amylase - breaks down starches, breads, and pasta.

Essential oils - Ginger, Myrrh, Cassia, Clary Sage, Canadian Fleabane

NOTE - Ashwagandha is not to be used if pregnant or nursing, trying to conceive, or have high cholesterol. Do not take if you are using blood glucose lowering medication. Some drug interactions may occur. Consult your doctor prior to use. Do not use this along with Thyromin™ or Thyroid medicine.

COMMENTS FROM YOUNG LIVING
"EndoGize™ is especially formulated to support a healthy and balanced endocrine system."

DIRECTIONS FOR USE
Take 1 capsule 2 times daily. Use daily for four weeks.
Discontinue for two weeks before resuming.

The statements about the supplement and the ingredients have not been evaluated by the Food and Drug Administration. Young Living® products are not intended to diagnose, treat, cure, or prevent any disease.

ESSENTIALZYME™

Essentialzyme™ is a good choice if you are looking for a broad spectrum digestive enzyme that also supports hormones. It is good for those who need help absorbing B12, Calcium, Iron, and Proteins. Essentialzyme™ should be used by people who have low stomach acid. It is the only enzyme supplement from Young Living® that contains Betaine HCL, which promotes the production of hydrochloric acid which is essential for high protein diets. This enzyme contains the most herbs.

INGREDIENTS
Total carbohydrate <1g (<1% DV)
Calcium (as di-calcium phosphate) 70 mg (6% DV)
Proprietary Blend (Light) 250 mg
  • Pancrelipase, Pancreatin, Trypsin
Proprietary Blend (Dark) 270mg
  • Betaine HCI, Bromelain
  • Thyme (Thymus vulgaris) leaf powder
  • Carrot (Daucus carota) root powder
  • Alfalfa (Medicago sativa) sprout powder
  • Alfalfa (Medicago sativa) leaf powder
  • Papain
  • Cumin (Cuminum cyminum) seed powder
  • Anise (Pimpinella anisum) seed oil
  • Fennel (Foeniculum vulgare) seed oil
  • Peppermint (Mentha piperita) leaf oil
  • Tarragon (Artemisia dracunculus) aerial parts oil
  • Clove (Syzygium aromaticum) bud oil

WHAT THE INGREDIENTS DO
  • Bromelain - breaks down meats, dairy, eggs, and grains, as well as seeds, nuts, leafy greens, and others. Supports blood to help with inflammation.
  • Papain - digestive aid, may help with parasites, shingles, diarrhea, and runny nose.
  • Betaine HCL (Betaine hydrochloride) - promotes the production of hydrochloric acid for digestion. Helps absorb B12, Calcium, Iron, and Proteins.
  • Pancrelipase - Good for poorly performing pancreas. Extract from pig pancreas.
  • Pancreatin (pancreas from pigs or cows) - helps produce other enzymes - Lipase, Protease, and Amylase . Good for those with a poorly performing pancreas.
  • Trypsin - breaks down proteins. For muscle growth and hormone production.
  • Digestive Supporting Herbs - Thyme, Carrot, Alfalfa sprout and leaf, and Cumin.
  • Digestive Supporting Oils - Anise, Fennel, Peppermint, Tarragon, and Clove.

COMMENTS FROM YOUNG LIVING
"Essentialzyme™ is a bilayered, multienzyme complex caplet specially formulated to support and balance digestive health and to stimulate overall enzyme activity to combat the modern diet. Essentialzyme™ contains Tarragon, Peppermint, Anise, Fennel, and Clove essential oils to improve overall enzyme activity, and support healthy pancreatic function."

DIRECTIONS FOR USE
Take 1 dual time-release caplet 1 hour before your largest meal of the day for best results.

The statements about the supplement and the ingredients have not been evaluated by the Food and Drug Administration. Young Living® products are not intended to diagnose, treat, cure, or prevent any disease.

ESSENTIALZYMES-4™

Essentialzymes-4™ helps support proper nutrient absorption. This is the broadest reaching Enzyme complex. If you don't know which digestive enzyme to choose, this is the one to get. It's dual release capsule ensures the proper break down of foods at the proper time during the digestive process. It contains bee pollen which is rich in antioxidants, vitamins, and minerals, as well as enzymes to help build your immune system and support brain function and alertness. This digestive enzyme also contains essential oils to help it become more bioavailable. This supplement is not vegan. Allerzyme™ is the only vegan enzyme.

INGREDIENTS
Total carbohydrate <1g (<1% DV)
Essentialzymes-4™ (White) Blend 225 mg
- Bee pollen powder
- Pancreatin
- Lipase
- Ginger (Zingibar officinale) root oil
- Fennel (Foeniculum vulgare) seed oil
- Tarragon (Artemisia dracunculus) leaf oil
- Anise (Pimpinella anisum) fruit oil
- Lemongrass (Cymbopogon flexuosus) leaf oil

WHAT THE INGREDIENTS DO
- Amylase - breaks down starch, breads, and pasta.
- Bromelain - breaks down meats, dairy, eggs, and grains, as well as seeds, nuts, leafy greens, and others. Supports blood to help with inflammation.
- Cellulase - breaks down man-made fiber, plant fiber, fruits, and veggies.
- Lipase - breaks down dietary fats and oils. Helps liver function.
- Phytase - helps with bone health and pulls needed minerals from grains.
- Protease 3.0 - supports circulation and toxicity. Higher acid to break down animal protein.
- Protease 4.5 - helps with sinusitis and has a lower acidic content.
- Protease 6.0 - helps with edema and carries away toxins. Least acidic.
- Papain - digestive aid, and may help parasites, shingles, diarrhea, and runny nose.
- Pancreatin (pancreas from pigs or cows) - helps produce other enzymes - amylase, lipase, and protease. Good for those with a poorly performing pancreas.
- Bee pollen - supports inflammation, a healthy immunity, menopause, and contains many vitamins, minerals, and antioxidants.
- Digestive Supporting Oils - Ginger, Fennel, Tarragon, Anise, Lemongrass, Rosemary.

COMMENTS FROM YOUNG LIVING
"Essentialzymes-4™ is a multi-spectrum enzyme complex specially formulated to aid the critically needed digestion of dietary fats, proteins, fiber, and carbohydrates commonly found in the modern processed diet. The dual time-release technology releases the animal- and plant-based enzymes at separate times within the digestive tract, allowing for optimal nutrient absorption."

DIRECTIONS FOR USE
Take 2 capsules (one dual dose blister pack) 2 times daily with largest meals.

The statements about the supplement and the ingredients have not been evaluated by the Food and Drug Administration. Young Living® products are not intended to diagnose, treat, cure, or prevent any disease.

FEMIGEN™

FemiGen™ supports a healthy libido, stress, energy, emotions, mood swings, vaginal dryness, PMS, hot flashes, appetite, fat burning, and is a natural alternative to estrogen therapy. Other herbs found in this supplement help boost your immunity and help aid digestion. One amino acid of note, L-cystine, is the basic building block of glutathione. Glutathione is a gem for longevity, liver detoxification, and cognitive health. With the added benefits of Iron and Magnesium for greater support with energy and immunity, FemiGen™ is a perfect supplement for hormonal changes.

INGREDIENTS
- Iron (4%)
- Magnesium (2%)
- Damiana (Turnera diffusa) leaf
- Epimedium (Epimedium sagittatum) aerial plant
- Wild yam (Dioscorea villosa) root
- Dong quai (Angelica sinensis) root
- Muira puama (Ptychopetalum olacoides) root
- American ginseng (Panax quinquefolius) root
- Licorice (Glycyrrhiza glabra) root extract
- Black cohosh (Cimicifuga racemosa) root
- L-carnitine
- Dimethylglycine HCl
- Cramp bark (Viburnum opulus) bark
- Squaw vine (Mitchella repens) aerial parts
- L-phenylalanine, L-cystine
- L-cysteine HCl
- Fennel (Foeniculum vulgare) seed oil
- Clary sage (Salvia sclarea) flowering top oil
- Sage (Salvia officinalis) leaf oil
- Ylang Ylang (Cananga odorata) flower oil

WHAT THE INGREDIENTS DO
- Damiana Leaf - supports libido, helps lower stress, healthy emotions and mood swings.
- Epimedium Aerial Plant (aka "Horny Goat Weed") - used to increase sexual drive.
- Wild Yam root (diosgenin) - natural alternative to estrogen therapy. Supports vaginal dryness, PMS, hot flashes, increased energy, and libido.
- Dong Quai root - helps ease menopausal symptoms and PMS.
- Muira puma root - increases sex drive, supports PMS, and can support joint pain.
- American ginseng root - supports stress, boosts immunity, and helps aid digestion.
- Licorice root extract - helps reduce stress and aids in digestion.
- Black cohosh root - helps ease menopause and PMS.
- L-carnitine - helps reduce lactic acid build up.
- Dimethylglycine HCL - helps improve the nervous system and immune system.
- Cramp Bark - helps with fluid retention, PMS and cramps.
- Squaw Vine aerial parts - supports peace, insomnia, menstruation, baby blues.
- L-phenylalanine - may help suppress appetite and help burn fat. Also helps with moods.
- L-cystine - building block of glutathione for oxidative stress, liver detoxification, and cognition.
- L-cysteine HCL - helps support anti-aging. Supports the immune system.
- Hormone supporting oils - Fennel, Clary Sage, Sage, Ylang Ylang

COMMENTS FROM YOUNG LIVING
"FemiGen™ capsules were formulated with herbs and amino acids designed to balance and support the female reproductive system from youth through menopause. FemiGen™ combines whole food herbs like wild yam, damiana, and dong quai, along with synergistic amino acids and select essential oils to supply nutrition that is supportive of the special needs of the female systems.

DIRECTIONS FOR USE
Take 2 capsules with breakfast and 2 capsules with lunch. When first starting out, use 1 capsule with breakfast and 1 capsule with lunch for 1-2 weeks. Monitor your body then increase to the recommended dose as needed.

ICP™

ICP™ is a part of Young Living's intestinal cleanse protocol. It is often joked that the ICP stands for "I see poo." It supports healthy digestion and a healthy colon.

INGREDIENTS

Iron 1 mg (2% DV)
ICP™ Blend 5 g

- Psyllium (Plantago ovata) seed powder
- Oat (Avena sativa) bran powder
- Flax (Linum usitatissimum) seed powder
- Fennel (Foeniculum vulgare) seed powder
- Rice (Oryza sativa) bran
- Guar (Cyamopsis tetragonoloba) gum seed powder
- Mojave yucca (Yucca schidigera) root
- Cellulose

- Fennel (Foeniculum vulgare) seed oil
- Anise (Pimpinella anisum) seed oil
- Tarragon (Artemisia dracunculus) leaf oil
- Aloe vera (Aloe barbadensis) leaf extract
- Ginger (Zingiber officinale) root oil
- Lemongrass (Cymbopogon flexuosus) leaf oil
- Rosemary (Rosmarinus officinalis) leaf oil
- Lipase

ICP™ Enzyme Blend 123 mg

- Lipase
- Protease 4.5, 3.0, and 6.0
- Phytase
- Peptidase

WHAT THE INGREDIENTS DO

- Iron - may improve muscle function, increase brain function and eliminate fatigue.
- Psyllium - helps constipation, digestion, blood sugar, cholesterol, and weight loss.
- Oat bran - aids digestion, regulates blood sugar levels, can help with weight loss.
- Flax seed - rich in dietary fiber, supports cholesterol, weight loss, and blood pressure.
- Fennel seed - improves digestion, lowers blood pressure, may promote weight loss.
- Rice bran - can aid in weight loss, may lower blood pressure and cholesterol levels.
- Guar gum seed - natural bonding agent.
- Mojave yucca root - may relieve pain and boosts the immune system.
- Cellulose - an important source of fiber.
- Fennel seed oil - improves digestion, lowers blood pressure, may promote weight loss.
- Anise seed oil - helps keep blood sugar levels stable, improves digestion.
- Tarragon leaf oil - improves digestion, fights bacteria.
- Aloe vera leaf extract - antioxidant and antimicrobial properties, can aid in digestion.
- Ginger root oil - improves digestion, reduces inflammation, improves liver function.
- Lemongrass leaf oil - supports the immune system, digestion, and cholesterol levels.
- Rosemary leaf oil - helps cleanse the liver, aids in digestion.

ICP™ Enzyme Blend 123 mg

- Lipase, Protease (4.5, 3.0, 6.0), Phytase, Peptidase - breaks down food for digestion and absorption.

COMMENTS FROM YOUNG LIVING

"ICP™ helps keep your colon clean with an advanced mix of fibers that scour out residues. A healthy digestive system is important for the proper functioning of all other systems because it absorbs nutrients that are used throughout the body. Enhanced with a special blend of essential oils, the fibers work to decrease the buildup of wastes, improve nutrient absorption, and help maintain a healthy heart."

DIRECTIONS FOR USE

Mix 2 rounded teaspoons with at least 8 oz. of juice or water. If cleansing or eating a high-protein diet, use 3 times daily. If eating a low-protein diet, use once daily. Drink immediately as this product tends to thicken quickly when added to liquid. Tastes best in juice or smoothies.

IMMUPRO™

ImmuPro™ helps strengthen the immune system and helps you fall asleep faster. Take one chewable tablet of ImmuPro™ about 30 minutes before bedtime. It has just the right amount of non-habit forming melatonin, because it is from a natural source, to help you drift off to dreamland and then it gets to work with its amazing ability to fight all that oxidative stress that you built up during the day. There are three powerhouse mushrooms in ImmuPro™. Reishi, maitake, and agaricus blazei mushrooms are delivered in powder form for some incredible benefits.

INGREDIENTS
- Strawberry (Fragaria chiloensis) fruit powder
- Wolfberry (Lycium barbarum) fruit polysaccharide
- Raspberry (Rubus idaeus) fruit powder
- Reishi (Ganoderma lucidum) whole mushroom powder
- Maitake Mushroom (Grifola frondosa) mycelia powder
- Arabinogalactan [from larch tree (larix laricina) wood extract]
- Mushroom (Agaricus blazei) mycelia powder
- Orange (Citrus sinensis) peel oil

Other Ingredients - Dextrose (non-GMO), Hydroxylproply cellulose, Stevia (Stevia rebaudiana). Silicon dioxide, Magnesium Stearate, Maltodextin (non-GMO)

WHAT THE INGREDIENTS DO
- Strawberry fruit powder - antioxidant and source of soluble and insoluble fiber.
- Wolfberry polysaccharides - known for their immune supporting and longevity benefits.
- Reishi mushroom - the Reishi mushroom is touted as the "king of herbs", and have been widely used in herbal medicine for their anti-aging properties. The polysaccharide content in these mushrooms are impressive and help to boost our immune system. The mushroom also supports the faster regeneration of healthy liver cells.
- Maitake mushroom - the maitake mushroom contains beta-glucan. According to the American Cancer Society, using beta-glucan is a powerful way to support the immune system. Beta-glucan works by activating macrophage cells, which are natural killer cells and T-cells.
- Agaricus blazei mushroom - agaricus blazei mushrooms also have beta-glucan and have been proven in multiple studies to help activate a normal healthy immune response. This mushroom in particular has also been studied and proven to help fight weight gain.
- Wolfberry and Larch Tree extracts - natural polysaccharides that support the healthy function of the immune system, as well as healthy regeneration of tissues and cells.

COMMENTS FROM YOUNG LIVING
"ImmuPro™ has been specially formulated to provide exceptional immune system support when combined with a healthy lifestyle and adequate sleep to support the body's needs. This power-packed formula combines naturally-derived immune-supporting NingXia wolfberry polysaccharides with a unique blend of reishi, maitake, and agaricus blazei mushroom powders to deliver powerful antioxidant activity to help reduce the damaging effects of oxidative stress from free radicals.

DIRECTIONS FOR USE
Directions - Take 1-2 chewable tablets at bedtime. Do not exceed 2 tablets per day. Cautions: contains Melatonin which may cause drowsiness. Do not drive or operate machinery while taking products containing Melatonin. Keep out of the reach of children.

The statements about the supplement and the ingredients have not been evaluated by the Food and Drug Administration. Young Living® products are not intended to diagnose, treat, cure, or prevent any disease.

INNER DEFENSE™

Inner Defense™ is an immunity boosting essential oil supplement. It is safe to consume daily, but can also be taken on days you are not feeling your best. Contrary to popular assumption, taking this daily will not upset your good gut flora. The oils in this capsule work in harmony with your gut, helping to strengthen your terrain, rather than beat it up. It is best to take Inner Defense™ as needed rather than on a daily basis. If you choose to take it at night before bed, do not take Life 9™ that night. Monitor your daily wellness and if you feel a little dip in your wellness, use Inner Defense™ as a one-time "bomb". This means you would take 1-2 capsules right when you need it at the very first signs of a wellness dip. If you choose to take it as a "bomb" at night, just before bed, then this will be the only capsules you will take. Skip Life 9™ for this nigt. Users who do this method report having a great night of sleep and wake up refreshed and fully back on track.

INGREDIENTS
Inner Defense™ 03 Super Blend 405 mg
- Virgin Coconut (Cocos nucifera) fruit oil
- Oregano (Origanum vulgare) leaf/stem oil
- Thyme (Thymus vulgaris) leaf oil
- Lemongrass (Cymbopogon flexuosus) leaf oil

Thieves® Essential Oil Blend 225 mg
Contains 13 drops total of Coconut carrier and pure essential oils.
- Clove (Syzygium aromaticum) bud oil
- Lemon (Citrus Limon) peel oil
- Eucalyptus radiata (Eucalyptus radiata) leaf oil
- Rosemary (Rosmarinus officinalis) leaf oil
- Cinnamon (Cinnamomum verum) bark oil

Other Ingredients - Fish gelatin, Glycerin, Water.
Note: Contains fish (tilapia, carp) and tree nuts (Coconut)

WHAT THE INGREDIENTS DO
- Coconut Oil - contains vitamins and minerals that support overall health.
- Oregano - rich in antioxidants and supports the immune system.
- Thyme - supports respiratory, digestive, immune and nervous systems, and mood.
- Lemongrass - known to boost a person's spirits. It is also used as an insect repellent.
- Clove - supports healthy microbial balance.
- Lemon - helps improve mental clarity and supports immunity.
- Eucalyptus - supports immunity, inflammation, and respiratory health.
- Rosemary - supports scalp and healthy hair. Supports cognition and immunity.
- Cinnamon Bark - supports immunity and respiratory systems.

COMMENTS FROM YOUNG LIVING
"Young Living's Inner Defense™ reinforces systemic defenses, creates unfriendly terrain for yeast/ fungus, promotes healthy respiratory function, and contains potent essential oils like Oregano, Thyme, and Thieves® which are rich in thymol, carvacrol, and eugenol for immune support. The liquid softgels dissolve quickly for maximum results. Softgel capsule has been reformulated with fish gelatin to remove the need for carrageenan and beeswax used in the porcine gelatin based softgel."

DIRECTIONS FOR USE
Take 1 softgel daily (a.m.) or take 1 softgel 3-5 times daily when needed.
For best results use Life 9™ eight hours later.

The statements about the supplement and the ingredients have not been evaluated by the Food and Drug Administration. Young Living® products are not intended to diagnose, treat, cure, or prevent any disease.

JUVAPOWER®

JuvaPower® is the supplement to take when you need extra help with alkalizing your body. It is a source of antioxidants and it supports your liver and helps to bind acids. JuvaPower® is an easy way to get added nutrients to support digestion, immunity, and cardiovascular health.

INGREDIENTS
- Rice (Oryza sativa) seed bran
- Spinach (Spinacia oleracea) leaf powder
- Tomato (Lycopersicon esculentum) fruit flakes
- Beet (Beta vulgaris) root powder
- Flaxseed (Linum usitatissumum) bran
- Oat seed (Avena sativa) bran
- Broccoli (Brassica oleracea) floret/stalk powder
- Cucumber (Cucumis sativus) fruit powder
- Dill (Anethum graveolens) seed
- Barley (Hordeum vulgare) sprouted seed
- Ginger (Zingiber officinale) root/rhizome powder
- Slippery elm (Ulmus fulva) bark
- Psyllium (Plantago ovata) seed husk
- Anise (Pimpinella anisum) seed
- Fennel (Foeniculum vulgare) seed
- Aloe vera (Aloe barbadensis) leaf extract
- Peppermint (Mentha piperita) leaf
- Anise (Pimpinella anisum) seed oil
- Fennel (Foeniculum vulgare) seed oil

WHAT THE INGREDIENTS DO
- Rice bran - can aid in weight loss, may lower blood pressure and cholesterol levels.
- Spinach (Spinacia oleracea) leaf powder - has beta-carotene, iron, and fiber providing benefits to support aging, immunity, digestion, and blood.
- Tomato fruit flakes - a good source of antioxidants and nutrients to support proper immune system functioning.
- Beet (Beta vulgaris) root powder - a health-promoting food that aids in increasing nitric oxide availability and can support hypertension and endothelial function.
- Flaxseed (Linum usitatissumum) bran - rich in alpha-linolenic acid (ALA, omega-3 fatty acids), lignans, and fiber that can support the cardiovascular and immune systems.
- Oat seed (Avena sativa) bran - a good source of B complex vitamins, vitamin E, protein, fat, minerals, and is rich in beta-glucan which is heart-healthy soluble fiber.
- Broccoli (Brassica oleracea) floret/stalk powder - an excellent source of vitamins K, E, C, B6, and A, phosphorus, potassium, magnesium, as well as folate and fiber.
- Cucumber (Cucumis sativus) fruit powder - has antioxidant, anti-inflammatory, and skin-conditioning properties.
- Dill (Anethum graveolens) seed - assists with relief of abdominal discomfort, colic, and digestion. It can also assist with ulcers, eye diseases, and uterine pains.
- Barley (Hordeum vulgare) sprouted seed - contains a variety of vitamins, minerals, and polyphenolic compounds that may improve cholesterol metabolism.
- Ginger (Zingiber officinale) root/rhizome powder - improves digestion, reduces inflammation, reduces cholesterol levels, and improves liver function.

- Slippery elm (Ulmus fulva) bark - supports common cold symptoms, supports digestion, urinary tract, and bowel.
- Psyllium (Plantago ovata) seed husk - stimulates the intestines to contract and helps speed the passage of stool through the digestive tract.
- Anise (Pimpinella anisum) seed and seed oil - helps keep blood sugar levels stable and improves digestion.
- Fennel (Foeniculum vulgare) seed and seed oil - improves digestion, helps move waste material out of the body, and is a mild appetite suppressant.
- Aloe vera (Aloe barbadensis) leaf extract - has antioxidant and antimicrobial properties, and can aid in digestion.
- Peppermint (Mentha piperita) leaf - increases energy and improves bowel movements.

COMMENTS FROM YOUNG LIVING

"JuvaPower® is a high antioxidant vegetable powder complex and is one of the richest sources of acid-binding foods. JuvaPower® is rich in liver-supporting nutrients and has intestinal cleansing benefits."

DIRECTIONS FOR USE

Sprinkle 7.5 grams (1 tablespoon) on food (i.e., baked potato, salad, rice, eggs, etc.) or add to 4-8 oz. purified water or rice/almond milk and drink. Use JuvaPower® three times daily for maximum benefits.

The statements about the supplement and the ingredients have not been evaluated by the Food and Drug Administration. Young Living® products are not intended to diagnose, treat, cure, or prevent any disease.

NOTES:

JUVATONE®

JuvaTone® is a liver supporting supplement and is helpful for those who tend to eat more animal protein. This supplement should be used when desiring to have optimal liver function. Whether you have had a bit too much to drink or you indulged in a meal high in animal protein, JuvaTone® is your go-to source! It is a powerful herbal supplement to support healthy liver function.

INGREDIENTS
- Calcium (dicalcium phosphate)
- Copper (copper citrate)
- Sodium

Proprietary JuvaTone® Blend
- Choline (C. bitarate)
- Dl-methionine
- Inositol
- Beet (Beta vulgaris) root
- Dandelion (Taraxacum officinale) root
- L-cysteine HCI
- Alfalfa (Medicago sativa) sprout
- Oregon grape (Berberis aquifolium) root
- Parsley (Petroselinum crispum) leaf powder
- Bee propolis
- Echinacea purpurea root

Proprietary Essential Blend
- Lemon (Citrus limon) peel oil
- German chamomile (Matricaria recutita) flower oil
- Geranium (Pelargonium graveolens) aerial parts oil
- Rosemary (Rosmarinus officinalis) leaf oil
- Myrtle (Myrtus communis) leaf oil
- Blue tansy (Tanacetum annuum) flowering top oil

Other Ingredients - Cellulose, Silicon dioxide, Magnesium stearate, Cellulose film-coating

WHAT THE INGREDIENTS DO
- Calcium (dicalcium phosphate) - helps prevent bone loss and repairs joints.
- Copper (copper citrate) - important in growth and development.
- Sodium - supports nerve impulses and maintains the balance of water and minerals.
- Choline (C. bitartrate) - supports metabolism, liver, and brain function.
- Dl-methionine - supports the liver, skin, hair, and strengthens nails, plus detoxes cells.
- Inositol - helps turn food into energy. Supports the immune system, hair and nails.
- Beet root (Beta vulgaris) - a health-promoting and disease-preventing functional food. Supports hypertension and endothelial function.
- Dandelion (Taraxacum officinale) root - a rich source of vitamin A. Supports the liver, gallbladder, bile ducts, and for minor digestive problems.
- L-cysteine HCI - supports glutathione levels for lung and brain function. Supports the liver.
- Alfalfa (Medicago sativa) sprout - a source of Vitamins A, C, E, and K4 and minerals calcium, potassium, phosphorous, and iron. Supports urinary system and cholesterol.
- Oregon grape (Berberis aquifolium) root - supports immunity and digestion.
- Parsley (Petroselinum crispum) leaf powder - improves digestion.

- Bee propolis - supports immunity.
- Echinacea purpurea root - supports immunity.
- Lemon (Citrus limon) peel oil - supports immune, digestive, and lymphatic systems.
- German chamomile (Matricaria recutita) flower oil - supports digestion and gas.
- Geranium (Pelargonium graveolens) aerial parts oil - anti-inflammatory properties.
- Rosemary (Rosmarinus officinalis) leaf oil - supports the liver and immunity.
- Myrtle (Myrtus communis) leaf oil - supports immunity.
- Blue tansy (Tanacetum annuum) flowering top oil - supports immunity and the liver.

COMMENTS FROM YOUNG LIVING

"JuvaTone® is a powerful herbal complex designed to promote healthy liver function. It is an excellent source of choline, a nutrient that is vital for proper liver function and necessary for those with high protein diets. JuvaTone® also contains inositol and dl-methionine, which helps with the body's normal excretion functions. Methionine also helps recycle glutathione, a natural antioxidant crucial for normal liver function. Other ingredients include Oregon grape root, a source of the liver-supporting compound berberine, and therapeutic-grade essential oils to enhance overall effectiveness."

DIRECTIONS FOR USE

Take 2 tablets 2 times daily. Increase as needed up to 4 tablets 4 times daily. Best when taken between meals.

The statements about the supplement and the ingredients have not been evaluated by the Food and Drug Administration. Young Living® products are not intended to diagnose, treat, cure, or prevent any disease.

NOTES:

K & B™

K & B™ is a liquid tincture that is a must for renal system support. The K and B stand for Kidney and Bladder. It supports the renal system to help increase urination and the liver to help support detoxification. It contains natural antioxidants and natural anti-inflammatory properties. K & B™ may be taken by adding to distilled water or added directly to veggie capsules.

INGREDIENTS
Proprietary K & B™ Blend - 3ml
- Juniper (Juniperus communis) berry extract
- Parsley (Petroselinum crispum) leaf extract
- Uva-ursi (Arctostaphylos uva-ursi) leaf extract
- Dandelion (Taraxacum officinale) root extract
- German chamomile (Matricaria recutita) flower extract
- Royal jelly
- Geranium (Pelargonium graveolens) aerial parts
- Fennel (Foeniculum vulgare) fruit
- Clove (Syzygium aromaticum) bud
- Roman chamomile (Chamaemelum nobile) aerial parts
- Sage (Salvia officinalis) aerial parts
- Juniper (Juniperus communis) branch/leaf/fruit

Other ingredients - Water, Ethanol alcohol

WHAT THE INGREDIENTS DO
- Juniper berry extract - supports digestion, intestinal gas, heartburn, bloating, and loss of appetite. Also supports the urinary tract, kidneys and bladder.
- Parsley leaf extract - supports the urinary tract, and gastrointestinal tract.
- Uva-ursi leaf extract - supports the urinary tract and painful urination.
- Dandelion root extract - supports digestion. Used to increase urine production and as a laxative to increase bowel movements. Rich in antioxidants. Supports liver health.
- German chamomile flower extract - supports digestion and gas.
- Royal jelly - produced by honey bees. Source of B vitamins. Supports the cardiovascular, kidneys, lungs, and immune systems.

Essential Oils -
- Geranium, Fennel, Clove, Roman chamomile, Sage, Juniper - supports digestion.

COMMENTS FROM YOUNG LIVING
"K & B™ is formulated to nutritionally support normal kidney and bladder health. It contains extracts of juniper berries, which enhance the body's efforts to maintain proper fluid balance; parsley, which supports kidney and bladder function and aids overall urinary health; and urva ursi, which supports both urinary and digestive system health. K & B™ is enhanced with therapeutic-grade essential oils."

DIRECTIONS FOR USE
Take 3 half droppers (3ml) three times daily in distilled water, or as needed.
Shake well before using.

The statements about the supplement and the ingredients have not been evaluated by the Food and Drug Administration. Young Living® products are not intended to diagnose, treat, cure, or prevent any disease.

KIDSCENTS® MIGHTYPRO™

KidScents® MightyPro™ is the perfect way to introduce prebiotics and probiotics to your little ones or even your big ones. The convenient single-serving packets make them the perfect travel companion. The over eight billion active cultures in MightyPro™ work to support your gut for a healthier immunity. They taste just like a "pixie stix" so everyone in your family is sure to become an instant fan. Just be sure not to let your fur babies have any. MightyPro™ contains xylitol, which can be toxic to dogs.

INGREDIENTS
Prebiotic blend
- Fructooligosaccharides, NingXia wolfberry (Lycium barbarum) fruit fiber

Probiotic strains
- Lactobacillus paracasei Lpc-37
- Lactobacillus acidophilus LA-14
- NingXia wolfberry (Lycium barbarum) fruit powder
- Lactobacillus plantarum LP-115
- Lactobacillus rhamnosus GG AF
- Streptococcus thermophilus
- Lactobacillus rhamnosus 6594
- Bifidobacterium infantis Bl-26

Other ingredients - Xylitol, Erythritol, Natural fruit punch flavor, Citric acid

WHAT THE INGREDIENTS DO
- Fructo-oligosaccharides (FOC) - food for gut flora.
- NingXia wolfberry (Lycium barbarum) fruit fiber - food for gut flora.
- Lactobacillus paracasei Lpc-37 - supports the digestive and immune system.
- Lactobacillus acidophilus LA-14 - has anti-inflammatory effects.
- NingXia wolfberry (Lycium barbarum) fruit powder - supports good bacteria in the gut.
- Lactobacillus plantarum LP-115 - inhibits the growth of pathogenic microorganisms.
- Lactobacillus rhamnosus GG AF - supports gastro-intestinal infections and immunity.
- Streptococcus thermophilus - breaks down lactose, supports digestion and immunity.
- Lactobacillus rhamnosus 6594 - supports a healthy gut and the immune system.
- Bifidobacterium infantis Bl-26 - improves digestion and the immune system.
- Xylitol - a natural sugar substitute from food.
- Erythritol - a natural zero-calorie sweetener for food.
- Natural fruit punch flavor - provides a sweet taste.
- Citric acid - it occurs naturally in citrus fruits and is a flavoring and preservative.

COMMENTS FROM YOUNG LIVING
"MightyPro™ is a unique, synergistic blend of prebiotics and probiotics in a supplement specially formulated for children. Packaged in easy, one-dose packets that can be taken almost anywhere you go, this supplement features over eight billion active, live cultures to support digestive and immune health."

DIRECTIONS FOR USE
For children 2 years and older, empty contents of 1 packet into mouth and allow to dissolve. Take 1 packet daily with food to provide optimal conditions for healthy gut bacteria. Can be combined with cold food or drinks. Do not add to warm or hot food or beverages.

The statements about the supplement and the ingredients have not been evaluated by the Food and Drug Administration. Young Living® products are not intended to diagnose, treat, cure, or prevent any disease.

KIDSCENTS® MIGHTYVITES™

KidScents® MightyVites™ are a chewable multi-vitamin that is perfect for your little ones. They contain vitamins, minerals, plant nutrients, and antioxidants to help support your child's healthy active lifestyle. MightyVites™ are also a great option for adults who have a hard time swallowing pills.

INGREDIENTS
Calories 25
Total Carbohydrates 5 g
Total Sugars 3 g
Includes 2 g Added Sugars
- Vitamin A (as beta carotene and from organic food blend) 180 mg
- Vitamin C (from organic food blend) 27 mg
- Vitamin D (as cholecalciferol) 5 mcg
- Vitamin E (from organic food blend) 30 mg
- Thiamin (from organic food blend) 0.8 mg
- Riboflavin (from organic food blend) 0.9 mg
- Niacin (from organic food blend) 9 mg
- Vitamin B6 (from organic food blend) 2.2 mg
- Folate (from organic food blend) 90 mcg DFE
- Vitamin B12 (from organic food blend) 3.2 mcg
- Biotin (from organic food blend) 40 mcg
- Pantothenic acid (from organic food blend) 1.8 mg
- Magnesium (from organic food blend) 4.5 mg
- Zinc (from organic food blend) 0.9 mg
- Selenium (from organic food blend) 4.5 mg

MightyVites™ Wild Berry Blend 97 mg
- Orgen-Kid Curry (murraya koenigii) leaf extract
- Guava (Psidium Guajava) fruit extract
- Lemon (Citrus limon) peel extract
- Sesbania (Sesbania grandiflora) leaf extract
- Amala (Phyllanthus emblica) fruit extract
- Holy Basil (Ocimum sanctum) aerial parts extract
- Annatto (Bixa orellana) seed extract
- Beet (Beta vulgaris) root juice powder
- Orange (Citrus sinensis) fruit juice powder
- Strawberry (Fragaria ananassa) fruit juice powder
- Wolfberry (Lycium barbarum) fruit powder
- Citrus flavonoids [from Tangerine (Citrus tangeria) peel]
- Barley grass (hordeum vulgare) leaf powder
- Broccoli (Brassica oleracea) sprout powder

Other Ingredients - Natural sweetener (Erythritol, Oligosaccharide), Malic acid, Stevia (Stevia rebaudiana) leaf extract, Silica, Magnesium Stearate

Orgen-Kid® contains the following natural food-based key ingredients - Natural mixed carotenoids, Natural vitamin B1 (Thiamin), Natural vitamin B2 (Riboflavin), Natural vitamin B3 (Niacin), Natural vitamin B5 (Pantothenate), Natural vitamin B6 (Pyridoxine), Natural vitamin B9 (Folate), Natural vitamin C, Natural vitamin E, Natural biotin, Natural magnesium, Natural zinc, Natural copper, Natural manganese, Natural potassium, Natural selenium, Wolfberry powder, Barley grass, Broccoli sprouts, Kosher vitamin D3, and Vitamin B12.

SUPPLEMENTS DESK REFERENCE

WHAT THE INGREDIENTS DO

- Vitamin A - protects the eyes and supports a healthy immune system.
- Vitamin C - supports cartilage, ligaments, tendons and skin. Helps healing.
- Vitamin D - helps maintain healthy bones, and supports a healthy immune system.
- Vitamin E - helps to prevent damage to cells.
- Thiamin - beneficial to a healthy nervous system.
- Riboflavin - needed for overall growth and supports energy levels.
- Niacin - supports circulation and cholesterol.
- Vitamin B6 - supports the immune system and supports moods.
- Folate - supports the heart.
- Vitamin B12 - is essential in red blood cell production and DNA synthesis.
- Biotin - is important for healthy skin and nails.
- Pantothenic acid - supports regeneration of the skin during wound healing.
- Magnesium - supports nerve and muscle functions, can help to prevent leg spasms.
- Zinc - helps growth and repair, supports immunity, hormones and digestion.
- Selenium - is a powerful antioxidant that defends against free radicals in the body.

MightyVites™ Wild Berry Blend

- Curry - helps with digestion and liver detoxification.
- Guava - supports good immunity and healthy digestion.
- Lemon - supports the body when cold symptoms occur.
- Sesbania - supports blood vessels to stay flexible.
- Amala - helps fend off free radicals which can cause aging.
- Holy Basil - helps to lower stress.
- Annatto - supports wound healing and healthy bones.
- Beet root juice - supports blood flow and may increase energy.
- Orange - has antioxidants that defend against free radicals.
- Strawberry - improves the skin and supports a healthy immune system.
- Wolfberry - supports eye health and overall health.
- Tangerine - supports eye health and reduces stress.
- Barley grass - is a detoxifier and natural antioxidant.
- Broccoli - is disease protection, supports a healthy immune system.

COMMENTS FROM YOUNG LIVING

KidScents® MightyVites™ include a full range of vitamins, minerals, antioxidants, and phytonutrients that deliver whole-food multinutrient support to your child's general health and well-being. Following in the footsteps of the recent Master Formula™ reformulation, MightyVites™ benefit from Orgen-kids®, a nutrient-dense, food-based superfruit, plant, and vegetable complex. Free of preservatives and artificial colors and flavors, these delicious, berry-flavored chewables give your children full nutritional support. Orgen-kids® is formulated with Orgen-FA®, which is the best source for natural folate available. Orgen-FA® is 100 percent USDA Certified Organic and does not contain synthetic folic acid or additives. It is extracted using hot water and is no different than the folic acid that is produced when boiling broccoli.

DIRECTIONS FOR USE

Children ages 4–12, take 4 chewable tablets daily.
Can be taken separately or in a single daily dose.

The statements about the supplement and the ingredients have not been evaluated by the Food and Drug Administration. Young Living® products are not intended to diagnose, treat, cure, or prevent any disease.

KIDSCENTS® MIGHTYZYME™

KidScents® MightyZyme™ chewables contain enzymes that naturally occur in the body that support and assist the digestive needs of growing bodies and the normal digestion of food.

INGREDIENTS
Calcium (from calcium carbonate) 50 mg (DV Kids <4yo 6%, >4yo 5%)
MightyZyme™ Blend 81 mg
- Lipase
- Alfalfa (Medicago sativa) leaf powder
- Amylase
- Protease 4.5
- Bromelain
- Carrot (Daucus carota sativa) root powder
- Peptidase
- Phytase
- Protease 6.0
- Protease 3.0
- Peppermint (Mentha Piperita) aerial parts oil
- Cellulase

Other Ingredients - Sorbitol, Dextrates, Natural mixed berry flavor, Microcrystalline cellulose, Magnesium stearate, Steric acid, Silica, Apple Juice powder, Stevia (Stevia rebaudiana) leaf extract

WHAT THE INGREDIENTS DO
- Calcium (from calcium carbonate) - supports bone, muscle, heart, and blood health.
- Lipase - breaks down dietary fats and oils. Helps liver function.
- Alfalfa leaf powder - for vitamins A, C, E, and K4, as well as minerals, calcium, potassium, phosphorus and iron.
- Amylase - breaks down starch, breads, and pasta.
- Protease 4.5 - helps with sinusitis and has a lower acidic content.
- Bromelain - breaks down meats, dairy, eggs, grains, and seeds and nuts.
- Carrot root powder - natural source of vitamin A, B, K, and potassium.
- Peptidase - finishes breaking down Proteases. Supports immunity and inflammation.
- Phytase - helps with bone health and pulls needed minerals from grains.
- Protease 6.0 - helps with edema and carries away toxins. Least acidic.
- Protease 3.0 - supports circulation and toxicity. Higher acid to break down animal protein.
- Peppermint oil - supports the healthy functioning of the digestive system.
- Cellulase - breaks down man-made fiber, plant fiber, fruits, and veggies.

Other Ingredients for flavor and formation - Sorbitol, Dextrates, Natural mixed berry flavor, Microcrystalline cellulose, Magnesium stearate, Steric acid, Silica, Apple Juice powder, Stevia leaf extract.

COMMENTS FROM YOUNG LIVING
"MightyZyme™ chewables contain enzymes that naturally occur in the body that support and assist the digestive needs of growing bodies and the normal digestion of foods."

DIRECTIONS FOR USE
Take 1 tablet 3 times daily prior to or with meals.
For relief of occasional symptoms including fullness, pressure, bloating, stuffed feeling (commonly referred to as gas), pain and/or minor cramping that may occur after eating.

The statements about the supplement and the ingredients have not been evaluated by the Food and Drug Administration. Young Living® products are not intended to diagnose, treat, cure, or prevent any disease.

LIFE 9™

Young Living® offers a synergy of nine different strains with 17 billion live active cultures in a delayed-release capsule to deliver the cultures directly to your intestines. Life 9™ is designed to give you the greatest possible benefits. It has nine strains to give you full-spectrum support, but what is interesting is that the best time to take it is at night just before bed or a few hours after dinner on an empty stomach. You should take this without any other supplement. Once you swallow it, it goes to work. All those beautiful healthy bacteria helping support your beautiful gut! It is said that 85% of all our issues stem from gut issues. You may take these every day or at least 3-4 times a week. This may also be used as a way to rapidly support your gut when you are feeling a dip in your immunity by consuming 5-6 at once right before bed. This is only to be done as needed and no more than once a month. Life 9™ will help to regulate your bowel movements. If you take too many for too long you may experience diarrhea. When you are having one bowel movement per full meal per day that is the right consistency, not too soft and not too hard, this means your gut is working correctly. There are no essential oils in Life 9™.

INGREDIENTS
- Lactobacillus acidophilus, Bifidobacterium lactis, Lactobacillus plantarum, Lactobacillus rhamnosus, Lactobacillus salivarius, Streptococcus thermophilus, Bifidobacterium breve, Bifidobacterium bifidum, Bifidobacterium longum

WHAT THE INGREDIENTS DO
- Lactobacillus acidophilus - antagonizes pathogens and has anti-inflammatory effects.
- Bifidobacterium lactis - breaks down waste, aids in absorption of vitamins and minerals.
- Lactobacillus plantarum - improves immune response, and supports IBS.
- Lactobacillus rhamnosus - promotes a healthy gut and supports the immune system.
- Lactobacillus salivarius - targets pathogenic bacteria; produces lactic acid that helps fight bad bacteria. Improves digestive health, immunity and dental health.
- Streptococcus thermophilus - helps break down lactose, supports digestion, and immunity.
- Bifidobacterium breve - competes with other bacteria, breaks down foods that are considered non-digestible; ferments sugars, produces lactic and acetic acids.
- Bifidobacterium bifidum - produces natural antibiotics that kill bad bacteria. Supports immunity and digestion.
- Bifidobacterium longum - Aids in normal digestion and balance of the intestinal tract.

COMMENTS FROM YOUNG LIVING
"Life 9™ is a proprietary, high-potency probiotic that combines 17 billion live cultures from nine beneficial bacteria strains that promotes healthy digestion, supports gut health, and helps maintain normal intestinal function for overall support of a healthy immune system. Life 9™ is specially designed with special delayed-release capsules, a dual-sorbent desiccant, and a special bottle and cap that ensure your Life 9™ stays fresh and effective. Each bottle contains 30 capsules, making it easy to use this helpful supplement daily."

DIRECTIONS FOR USE
Take 1 capsule every night following a meal or as needed.
REFRIGERATE AFTER OPENING.

LONGEVITY™

Longevity™ softgels are a pre-mixed essential oil synergy that is ready to consume. The best part is they come in thick walled capsules that are designed to dissolve in your intestines rather than your stomach. This is important because getting oils into your intestines promotes better health than allowing your stomach acids to come in contact with the oils. While stomach acid is not a huge offense to oils, there are some added benefits to getting them into your intestines rather than your digestive system. Supporting your gut goes a long way toward longevity!

INGREDIENTS
- Medium chain triglycerides (from fractionated Coconut oil)
- Coconut (Cocos nucifera) fruit oil
- Thyme (Thymus vulgaris) leaf oil
- Orange (Citrus sinensis) peel oil
- Clove (Syzygium aromaticum) flower bud oil
- Frankincense (Boswellia carterii) gum/resin oil

Contains 14 drops total of Coconut carrier and pure essential oils.
Other ingredients - Hypromellose, Water, Silica, Mixed tocopherols (vitamine E)
Note: Contains tree nuts (Coconut)

WHAT THE INGREDIENTS DO
- Medium chain triglycerides (from fractionated Coconut oil) - beneficial for cognitive function, mood balance and weight management; assists in digestion and nutrient absorption; heart protective with antioxidant properties.
- Coconut fruit oil - enhances immunity and digestion; beneficial for brain, heart and oral health; protective for kidneys, liver and urinary tract; assists with energy production.
- Thyme leaf oil - beneficial for immune, respiratory, digestive and nervous systems; assists in cognitive function, hormone balance and relaxation; assists with oral, eye and skin health.
- Orange peel oil - enhances immunity, improves blood flow and assists a healthy blood pressure; helps to fight signs of aging in skin and promotes the production of collagen.
- Clove flower bud oil - high in antioxidants; boosts the immune system, assists in oral, digestive and cardiovascular health and is protective for the liver.
- Frankincense gum/resin oil - immune enhancing and stress reducing; beneficial for skin health and to fight signs of aging; assists in hormone balance, cognitive function, digestion and sleep.

COMMENTS FROM YOUNG LIVING
"Longevity™ softgels are a potent, proprietary blend of fat-soluble antioxidants. Longevity™ blend should be taken daily to strengthen the body's systems to prevent the damaging effects of aging, diet, and the environment. Enriched with the pure essential oils Thyme, Orange, and Frankincense. Longevity™ protects DHA levels, a nutrient that supports brain function and cardiovascular health, promotes healthy cell regeneration, and supports liver and immune function. Longevity™ also contains clove oil, nature's strongest antioxidant, for ultra antioxidant support."

DIRECTIONS FOR USE
Take 1 softgel capsule once daily with food or as needed.

The statements about the supplement and the ingredients have not been evaluated by the Food and Drug Administration. Young Living® products are not intended to diagnose, treat, cure, or prevent any disease.

MASTER FORMULA™

If you want to choose an "All Star" for daily supplementation, Master Formula™ would be the winner. It is a three part daily supplement designed to support your full health spectrum. To highlight some of its amazing qualities, it contains ALL B vitamins, vegan vitamin D3, and gut supporting pre-biotics. It contains the coveted Turmeric Root Essential Oil, which is loaded with antioxidants and amazing for glowing skin and hair. Even though Young Living® does not sell this as a single oil, it is great to know you can get its benefits through using Master Formula™! The Calcium it contains is Calcium Ascorbate which is a more gentle form of calcium for those with sensitive tummies. Master Formula™ also contains 60% of your daily iron needs and the vitamin K2 for bone and heart health. This supplement is packed full of herbs and veggies that have been juiced and dried to deliver pure phytonutrients from plants that have been picked at the peak of harvest.

INGREDIENTS
- A (Beta-carotene) 100% DV
- B1 (Thiamin) 730% DV
- B2 (Riboflavin) 590% DV
- B3 (Niacin) 90% DV
- B5 (Pantothenic acid) 190% DV
- B6 (Pyridoxine) 550% DV
- B7 (Biotin or Vitamin H) 100% DV
- B9 (Folate. NOT Folic Acid) 90% DV
- B12 (Methylcobalamin) 200% DV
- C (Calcium Ascorbate and acerola cherry) 100% DV
- D3 (Cholecalciferol) 100% DV
- E 170% DV
- K2 60% DV
- Calcium Carbonate 20% DV
- Chromium 100% DV
- Copper 20% DV
- Iron 60% DV
- Magnesium 15% DV
- Manganese 100% DV
- Molybdenum 100% DV
- Potassium <2%
- Selenium (amino acid) 110% DV
- Zinc 100% DV
- Choline bitartrate (this is not B4 as some assume)
- Probiotics (Wolfberry Fiber and Fructooligosaccharides)
- Probiotics (Wolfberry Fiber)

Proprietary Master Formula Tablet Blend 208 mg
Choline bitartrate, Fructooligosaccharides, Trace minerals
Proprietary Master Formula Essential Oil Blend 7.5 mg
Turmeric (Curcuma longa) root oil, Cardamom (Elettaria cardamomum) fruit/seed oil, Clove (Syzygium aromaticum) flower bud oil, Fennel (Foeniculum vulgare) seed oil, Ginger (Zingiber officinale) root oil

Proprietary Master Formula Capsule Blend 42 mg
Atlantic kelp, Inositol, PABA (Para amino benzoic acid), Spirulina algae, Barley grass, Citrus bioflavonoids [from Lemon (Citrus limon) whole fruit powder, Orange (Citrus sinensis) whole fruit powder, Lime (Citrus aurantifolia) whole fruit powder, Tangerine (Citrus reticulata) whole fruit powder, Grapefruit (Citrus paradisi) whole fruit powder], Orange (Citrus sinensis) fruit powder, NingXia wolfberry (Lycium barbarum) fruit powder, Olive (Olea europaea) leaf extract, Boron citrate, Lycopene

Spectra™ Fruit, Vegetable, and Herb Blend 100mg
Coffea arabica fruit extract, Broccoli (Brassica oleracea italica) seed concentrate, Camellia sinensis leaf extract, Onion (Allium cepa) bulb extract, Apple (Malus domestica) fruit skin extract, Acerola (Malpighia glabra) fruit extract, Camu-camu (Myrciaria dubia) fruit concentrate, Japanese saphora (Sophora japonica) flower extract, Tomato (Lycopersicon esculentum) fruit concentrate, Broccoli (Brassica oleraca italica) floret and stem concentrate, Cabbage palm (Euterpe oleracea) fruit concentrate, Turmeric (Curcuma longa) root concentrate, Garlic (Allium sativum) clove concentrate, Basil (Ocimum basilicum) leaf concentrate, Oregano (Origanum vulgare) leaf concentrate, Cassia (Cinnamomum cassia) branch/stem concentrate, European elder (Sambucus nigra) fruit concentrate, Carrot (Daucus carota sativa) root concentrate, Mangosteen (Garcinia mangostana) fruit concentrate, Black currant (Ribes nigrum) fruit extract, Blueberry (Vaccinium angustifolium) fruit extract, Sweet cherry (Prunus avium) fruit concentrate, Blackberry (Rubus fruticous) fruit concentrate, Chokeberry (Aronia melanocarpa) fruit concentrate, Raspberry (Rubus idaeus) fruit concentrate, Spinach (Spinacia oleracea) leaf concentrate, Collards (Brassica oleracea acehala) leaf concentrate, Bilberry (Vaccinium myrtillus) fruit extract, Brussels sprout (Brassica oleracea gemmifera) head concentrate

Other Ingredients: Sunflower lecithin (non-GMO), Hypromellose, Magnesium stearate (vegetable source), Silicon dioxide, Microcrystalline cellulose, Stearic acid, Croscarmellose sodium, Organic maltodextrin, Silicon dioxide, Organic palm olein, Organic guar gum.

WHAT THE INGREDIENTS DO
- A (Beta-carotene) - supports vision, immunity, and overall health.
- B1 (Thiamin) - enables the body to use carbohydrates as energy.
- B2 (Riboflavin) - helps break down proteins, fats, and carbohydrates into energy
- B3 (Niacin) - helps lower cholesterol, ease arthritis and boost brain function.
- B5 (Pantothenic acid) - necessary for making blood cells, converts food into energy.
- B6 (Pyridoxine) - creates red blood cells.
- B7 (Biotin or Vitamin H) - supports a healthy metabolism and creates enzymes.
- B9 (Folate. NOT Folic Acid) - plays a crucial role in cell growth.
- B12 (Methylcobalamin) - supports the body to make red blood cells.
- C (Calcium Ascorbate and acerola cherry) - boosts immunity.
- D3 (Cholecalciferol) - helps your body absorb calcium and phosphorus, strong bones.
- E - antioxidant, helps to protect cells from the damage caused by free radicals.
- K2 - metabolizes calcium, the main mineral found in your bones and teeth.
- Calcium Carbonate - for healthy bones, muscles, nervous system, and heart.
- Chromium - improves insulin sensitivity, enhances protein, carbohydrate, and lipid metabolism.
- Copper - supports red blood cells and maintains nerve cells and the immune system.
- Iron - supports healthy blood and immunity; may support fatigue.
- Magnesium - regulates muscle and nerve function, blood sugar levels, and blood pressure.
- Manganese - helps activate many enzymes in metabolism.
- Molybdenum - removes toxins from the metabolism of sulfur containing amino acids.
- Potassium - helps regulate muscle contractions, supports nerve function and fluid balance.
- Selenium (amino acid) - antioxidant properties.
- Silicon - stimulates the rapid regrowth of damaged skin tissue.
- Zinc - helps the immune system fight off invading bacteria and viruses.

Proprietary Master Formula Tablet Blend
- Choline bitartrate (this is not B4 as some assume) - supports brain memory.
- Prebiotics (Wolfberry Fiber and Fructooligosaccharides) - food for good gut flora.

Proprietary Master Formula Essential Oil Blend
- Turmeric root oil, Cardamom fruit/seed oil, Clove flower bud oil, Fennel seed oil, Ginger root oil - supports immunity and bioavailability of herbs.

Proprietary Master Formula Capsule Blend
- Atlantic kelp - rich source of iodine.
- Inositol - helps turn food into energy. Supports the immune system, hair, and nails.
- PABA (Para amino benzoic acid) - supports skin elasticity, hair loss and color, and joints.
- Spirulina algae- supports blood lipids, blood sugar, and blood pressure.
- Barley grass - supports digestion and helps reduce constipation.
- Citrus bioflavonoids (whole fruit powders) - supports immunity and oxidative stress.
- Olive (Olea europaea) leaf extract - supports the brain and heart.
- Boron citrate - supports bones, muscles, testosterone levels, and mental clarity.
- Lycopene - supports antioxidative stress and heart health.

Spectra™ Fruit, Vegetable, and Herb Blend
- Coffea arabica fruit extract - antioxidants known to protect brain cells.
- Broccoli seed concentrate - detoxification to support brain and increases glutathione.
- Camellia sinensis leaf extract - aka green tea - supports oxidative stress.
- Onion bulb extract - high in vitamins, minerals, and antioxidants.
- Apple fruit skin extract - supports digestion and cardiovascular health.
- Acerola fruit extract - high in vitamin C, supports immune health.
- Camu-camu fruit concentrate - high in vitamin C and antioxidants.
- Japanese sophora flower extract - has anti-oxidative and anti-inflammatory activities.
- Tomato fruit concentrate - source of vitamin C, potassium, folate, and vitamin K.
- Broccoli floret and stem concentrate - vitamins K, A, C, calcium, phosphorus, and zinc.
- Cabbage palm fruit concentrate - high in vitamin C and K.
- Turmeric root concentrate - antioxidants that support heart disease, memory, and mood.
- Garlic clove concentrate - antioxidants that support the brain, blood, and cells.
- Basil leaf concentrate - supports stress, and has anti-inflammatory and antioxidant properties.
- Oregano leaf concentrate - antioxidant and antibacterial.
- Cassia branch/stem concentrate - supports renal, circulatory, and immune systems.
- European elder fruit concentrate - antioxidants that support heart health, immunity, and stress.
- Carrot root concentrate - good source of vitamin A and antioxidants to support blood.
- Mangosteen fruit concentrate - antioxidants; supports skin, immunity, and blood sugar.
- Black currant fruit extract - high in vitamin C, antioxidants for skin and anti-aging.
- Blueberry fruit extract - high in nutrients and antioxidants to support blood and cells.
- Sweet cherry fruit concentrate - supports joints, muscles, brain, sleep, and immunity.
- Blackberry fruit concentrate - high in antioxidants, vitamins C, K, and A.
- Chokeberry fruit concentrate - high in phenols, supports immunity.
- Raspberry fruit concentrate - antioxidants that support heart health and circulation.
- Spinach leaf concentrate - supports blood; high in calcium, folic acid, and vitamins A and C.
- Collards leaf concentrate - high in folate, calcium, and vitamins E, A, K, and C.
- Bilberry fruit extract - supports blood vessels, cellular health, and circulation.
- Brussels sprout head concentrate - antioxidants that support cells; high in vitamin K.

COMMENTS FROM YOUNG LIVING
"Master Formula™ is a full spectrum, multinutrient complex, providing premium vitamins, minerals, and food-based nutriment to support general health and well-being. By utilizing a Synergistic Suspension Isolation process – SSI Technology – ingredients are delivered in three distinct delivery forms. Collectively, these ingredients provide a premium, synergistic complex to support your body."

BENEFITS
- Naturally supports general health and well-being for the body
- Gut flora supporting prebiotics
- Ingredients help neutralize free radicals in the body
- Includes antioxidants, vitamins, minerals, and food-based nutriment
- Pre-packaged sachets are convenient to take your vitamins on the go
- SSI Technology delivers ingredients in three forms chosen for their complementary properties

MICRONIZED NUTRIENT CAPSULE
This capsule supports the body naturally through lycopene, wolfberry powder, and citrus bioflavonoids. The capsule also contains Orgen-B®, which is a blend of certified organic guava, mango, and lemon extracts for a perfect synergy of B vitamins and chelated minerals. It contains 100% natural vitamin B1, B2, B3, B5, B6, and B9. Orgen Family® states, "B-vitamins help critically with a range of normal body functions, from cellular growth to metabolism. Vitamin B3, also known as Niacin, helps in the metabolism of glucose and fat. Vitamin B6, also known as pyridoxine, dominates the metabolism of amino acids and lipids. Vitamin B9 acts as a coenzyme in the form of folates that aids the production of red blood cells."

PHYTO-CAPLET
Contains trace minerals and gut flora-supporting prebiotics. Phyto-caplet also contains Spectra™, a powerful antioxidant that contains fruit, veggie, and herb extracts with Vitamin C. FutureCeuticals, Inc. states, "Spectra™ represents the latest evolution in the fight against potentially-damaging free radicals. For the first time anywhere, the biological effects of a natural supplement on the changes of oxidative and nitrosative stress markers, as well as cellular metabolic activity, have been clinically observed in the human body. Exclusively available from FutureCeuticals, Spectra™ has been reported to decrease ROS, increase cellular oxygen consumption in blood and mitochondria, decrease extracellular $H2O2$, and reduce TNFa-induced inflammatory response in humans."

LIQUID VITAMIN CAPSULE
Contains Cardamom, Clove, Fennel, and Ginger essentials oils. The Liquid Vitamin Capsule also contains turmeric root oil, a powerfully oxygenating oil that supports overall health. This capsule contains fat soluble vitamins A, E, K, and a vegan sourced vitamin D3. These all provide excellent antioxidant support.

DIRECTIONS FOR USE
Take 1 packet (1 liquid capsule, 1 caplet, 2 capsules) daily with water.

MEGACAL™

MegaCal™ was formulated to help support the body's calcium needs. It contains a synergistic blend of multiple calciums, along with magnesium, manganese, and vitamin C to support cell health and proper bone formation and maintenance. MegaCal™ is a powdered formula to be mixed with water or juice for proper calcium absorption.

INGREDIENTS
- Vitamin C
- Calcium (lactate, glycerophosphate, carbonate, and ascorbate)
- Magnesium (as citrate, sulfate, and carbonate)
- Manganese (as sulfate)

Proprietary MegaCal ™ Blend -
- Xylitol
- Lemon (Citrus Limon) rind oil

Other Ingredient - Fractionated Coconut oil

WHAT THE INGREDIENTS DO
- Vitamin C - antioxidant that supports cartilage, ligaments, tendons and skin. Helps healing.
- Calcium lactate - supports calcium deficiencies.
- Calcium glycerophosphate - supports calcium and phosphorus levels.
- Calcium carbonate - added calcium for healthy bones, muscles, heart, and nervous system.
- Calcium ascorbate - a form of vitamin C that contains 10% absorbable calcium.
- Magnesium (as citrate, sulfate, and carbonate) - important for bone formation and calcium absorption; important for carbohydrate and glucose metabolism; helps maintain muscle health and heart health; helps reduce muscle tension.
- Manganese (as sulfate) - essential for bone development and maintenance; promotes normal functioning of the brain, nervous system and enzyme systems; protects against free radicals; promotes healthy blood sugar levels.

Proprietary MegaCal ™ Blend -
- Xylitol - sugar substitute.
- Lemon rind oil - promotes skin health, aids in weight loss efforts, improves bone density.

Other Ingredient - Fractionated coconut oil - source of quick energy; helps improve insulin sensitivity; may assist in weight loss.

COMMENTS FROM YOUNG LIVING
"MegaCal™ is a wonderful source of calcium, magnesium, manganese, and vitamin C. MegaCal™ supports normal bone and vascular health as well as normal nerve function and contains 207 mg of calcium and 188 mg of magnesium per serving."

DIRECTIONS FOR USE
Take 1 scoop (1 tsp) (5g) with 1 cup (240 ml) of water or juice daily, one hour after a meal or taking medication or an hour before bedtime. Do not exceed 3 servings daily. DO NOT FEED TO DOGS.

The statements about the supplement and the ingredients have not been evaluated by the Food and Drug Administration. Young Living® products are not intended to diagnose, treat, cure, or prevent any disease.

MINDWISE™

MindWise™ is formulated to help healthy brain function. It supports cardiovascular health for better cognition. Antioxidants support immunity and proper cell function. Taken on a regular basis, MindWise™ is a smart choice for a healthy heart and mind. It comes in two packages: as a serum to be taken by the spoonful, and in single-serving sachets for easy storing and use.

INGREDIENTS
- Vitamin D (as D3)

Proprietary Memory Blend – 378.4 mg
- Pomegranate fruit extract
- Rhododendron leaf extract
- L-alpha glycerylphosphorylcholine (GPC)
- Acetyl-L-Carnitine (ALCAR)
- Coenzyme Q10 (31.8 mg per serving)
- Turmeric root powder

Proprietary Oil Blend – 397.4 mg
- Sacha inchi seed oil, Medium chain triglycerides, Essential Oils - Lemon, Peppermint, Fennel, Anise, Lime.

Other Ingredients - Water, Pomegranate juice concentrate, Acai puree, Glycerin, Sunflower lecithin, Natural flavors, Malic acid, Citric acid, Luo han guo fruit extract, No preservatives

WHAT THE INGREDIENTS DO
- Vitamin D (D3) - supports mood, healthy bones, and immunity.
- Pomegranate fruit extract - high antioxidant benefits.
- Rhododendron leaf extract - beneficial polyphenols and flavonoids.
- L-alpha glycerylphosphorylcholine (GPC) - builds cell membranes and contributes to the production of neurotransmitters.
- Acetyl-L-Carnitine (ALCAR) - antioxidant that supports normal brain function.
- Coenzyme Q10 - helps produce energy, normal growth, maintenance and repair.
- Turmeric root powder - promotes healthy inflammation in the body.
- Sacha inchi seed oil - vegetarian oil supports healthy brain and cardiovascular health.
- Medium chain triglycerides - supports cardiovascular health and cognitive function.
- Essential oils - supports absorption of other ingredients; high in antioxidants.
- Pomegranate juice - adds flavor and high in antioxidants.
- Acai puree - adds flavor and high in antioxidants.
- Luo Han Guo - adds sweetness with no calories (Monk fruit).
- Sunflower lecithin - rich in choline - beneficial to brain health.
- Glycerin - adds base and sweet taste.
- Malic acid - found in apples and pears; supports energy.

COMMENTS FROM YOUNG LIVING

"Support normal cardiovascular health and cognitive health with the fruity, nutty flavor of MindWise™! With a vegetarian oil made from cold-pressed sacha inchi seeds harvested from the Peruvian Amazon and other medium-chain triglyceride oils, MindWise™ has a high proportion of unsaturated fatty acids and omega-3 fatty acids. Plus, it uses a combination of fruit juices and extracts, turmeric, and pure essential oils to create a heart and brain function supplement with a taste you'll love! MindWise™ also includes our proprietary memory function blend made with bioidentical CoQ10, ALCAR, and GPC—ingredients that have been studied for their unique benefits. With generous amounts of vitamin D3, this premium supplement is equipped to support normal brain function and overall cognitive and cardiovascular health."

BENEFITS

- Supports normal brain and heart function
- Contains a high proportion of unsaturated fatty acids and omega-3 fatty acids
- Includes beneficial GPC, ALCAR, and bioidentical CoQ10
- Supports heart health by replenishing the body with CoQ10
- Features an improved, smoother texture
- Includes no added preservatives
- Formulated with turmeric

DIRECTIONS FOR USE

16 oz Bottle -
Take 1 tablespoon (3 teaspoons) once daily.
Children (4+ years) should take 1–2 teaspoons once daily.
Should be taken with a meal.
Shake well before each use.
Consume within 30 days of opening.

Single-Serve Packet -
Drink 1 sachet daily.
Consume promptly after opening.
Should be taken with a meal.
Shake well before use.

- For optimal effect adults should follow initial dose schedule for 7-10 days followed by maintenance schedule.
- Children (4-12) should follow children's schedule (see above under 16 oz. Bottle).
- If you are pregnant, nursing, taking medication, or have a medical condition, consult a health care professional prior to use.
- Should be taken with a meal. Shake well before use. Refrigerate after opening.

The statements about the supplement and the ingredients have not been evaluated by the Food and Drug Administration. Young Living® products are not intended to diagnose, treat, cure, or prevent any disease.

MINERAL ESSENCE™

We often find ourselves depleted of the vital minerals we need every day. This powerful, fully balanced mineral tincture is the perfect way to supplement our growing mineral needs. Shake this well before using. You can add the 5mls needed to five 00 capsules or simply add it to 4-8 ounces of water.

INGREDIENTS
Calories per serving - 10
Carbohydrates 3 g (DV <1%)
Sugars 2 g
Includes 2 g Added Sugars (DV 3%)
Magnesium - 350 mg (DV 80%)
Chloride - 1,000 mg (DV 45%)
Sodium - 3 g (DV <1%)
Mineral Essence™ Blend – 5ml
- Salt (trace mineral complex)
- Honey
- Royal Jelly
- Lemon (Citrus limon) peel oil
- Cinnamon (Cinnamomum verum) Bark oil
- Peppermint (Mentha piperita) aerial parts oil

WHAT THE INGREDIENTS DO
- Magnesium - supports bone formation, calcium absorption, carbohydrate and glucose metabolism, muscle health, and heart health.
- Chloride - supports blood volume and pressure. Supports fluid balance in cells.
- Sodium - supports nerve impulses and maintains the balance of water and minerals.

Mineral Essence™ Blend – 5ml
- Salt - supports nerve impulses and maintains the balance of water and minerals.
- Honey - antioxidant that supports immunity, digestion, heart, and gut health.
- Royal Jelly - produced by honey bees. Source of B vitamins. Supports the cardiovascular, kidneys, lungs, and immune systems.
- Lemon peel oil - natural detoxifier, promotes weight loss, boosts immune system and energy.
- Cinnamon Bark oil - supports healthy immunity, circulation, digestion and energy.
- Peppermint oil - supports healthy digestion, immunity, energy, and brain health.

COMMENTS FROM YOUNG LIVING
"Mineral Essence™ is a balanced, full-spectrum ionic mineral complex enhanced with essential oils. According to two time Nobel Prize winner Linus Pauling PhD. "You can trace every sickness, every disease, and every ailment to a mineral deficiency." Ionic minerals are the most fully and quickly absorbed form of minerals available."

DIRECTIONS FOR USE
Take 5 half-droppers (1ml each) morning and evening or as needed as a mineral supplement. May be added to 4-8 oz. of distilled/purified water or juice before drinking. This product contains royal jelly, which may cause allergic reactions. Shake well before using and refrigerate after opening.

The statements about the supplement and the ingredients have not been evaluated by the Food and Drug Administration. Young Living® products are not intended to diagnose, treat, cure, or prevent any disease.

MULTIGREENS™

MultiGreens™ is the perfect daily pairing to NingXia Red® for overall health support. It is rich in antioxidants to support healthy cell function. MultiGreens™ supports healthy memory, mood, and other nervous system functions. It contains sea kelp, which is a great source of minerals, most notably, iodine. It also contains spirulina, which is an excellent source of bioavailable calcium, niacin, potassium, magnesium, iron, and B vitamins. Use MultiGreens™ daily for best results.

INGREDIENTS
- Bee pollen
- Barley (Hordeum vulgare) grass juice concentrate
- Spirulina (Spirulina platensis)
- Choline (as choline bitartrate)
- Eleuthero (Eleutherococcus senticosus) root
- Alfalfa (Medicago sativa) stem/leaf extract
- Kelp (Laminaria digitata) whole thallus
- Amino Acid Complex (L-Arginine, L-Cysteine, L-Tyrosine)

MultiGreens™ oil blend - Rosemary (Rosmarinus officinalis) leaf oil, Lemon (Citru limon) peel oil, Lemongrass (Cymbopogon flexuosus) leaf oil, Melissa (Melissa officinalis) leaf/flower oil)

Other ingredients - Gelatin, Silica (capsule and substrate).

WHAT THE INGREDIENTS DO
- Bee pollen - antioxidants that protect against free radicals in the body.
- Barley grass juice concentrate - source of minerals; improves digestive function.
- Spirulina - contains calcium, niacin, potassium, magnesium, B vitamins and iron.
- Choline - supports brain memory, mood, muscle control, and nervous system functions.
- Eleuthero root - helps the body better adapt to stress; supports nervous system function.
- Alfalfa stem/leaf extract - supports healthy cholesterol and glucose levels.
- Kelp - supports metabolism. Sea kelp is the richest natural source of iodine.

MultiGreens™ oil blend -
- Rosemary leaf oil - supports hair growth, mental acuity, and respiratory function.
- Lemon peel oil - cleanses toxins from the body and stimulates lymphatic drainage.
- Lemongrass leaf oil - supports immunity and circulatory systems.
- Melissa leaf/flower oil - is used as a digestive aid.

Amino Acid Complex -
- L-arginine - supports blood and circulation.
- L-cysteine - supports metabolism and energy.
- L-tyrosine - supports nerve cell communication and may support moods.

COMMENTS FROM YOUNG LIVING
"MultiGreens™ is a nutritious chlorophyll formula designed to boost vitality by working with the glandular, nervous, and circulatory systems. MultiGreens™ is made with spirulina, alfalfa sprouts, barley grass, bee pollen, eleuthero, Pacific kelp, and therapeutic-grade essential oils."

DIRECTIONS FOR USE
If you have a slow metabolism, take 3 capsules two times daily. If you have a fast metabolism, take 4 capsules once or twice daily. Best taken 1 hour before meals. For stomach sensitivity, take with meals.

The statements about the supplement and the ingredients have not been evaluated by the Food and Drug Administration. Young Living® products are not intended to diagnose, treat, cure, or prevent any disease.

NINGXIA RED®

NingXia Red® is a powerhouse of antioxidants and nutrients that the whole family will benefit from using. It is a whole body supplement for a more healthful life experience. The wolfberry, also known as the goji berry, is touted for having high antioxidant properties. A daily shot helps support better energy and normal cellular function, as well as whole-body health and wellness. Four ounces of NingXia Red® equals one serving of fruit; however, one ounce has the antioxidant equivalent to eating four pounds of carrots or eight whole oranges! NingXia Red® is safe for all people from solid-food eating children to adults. Pregnant and nursing women should also consider using NingXia Red® as part of their healthy daily regimen. The Orange, Yuzu, Lemon, and Tangerine essential oils in NingXia Red® contain d-limonene, which is a powerful wellness-promoting constituent. NingXia Red® is free of high fructose sweeteners. Wolfberries and exotic fruits such as blueberry, cherry, aronia, pomegranate, and plum give NingXia Red® its delicious flavor.

INGREDIENTS
2 oz per serving
Calories per serving - 25
Carbohydrates 6 g (DV 2%)
Sugars 5 g
Protein - <1 g
- Calcium - 40 mg (DV 4%)
- Iron - 0.4 mg (DV 2%)
- Sodium - 35 mg (DV 2%)

Proprietary NingXia Red® Blend - 58 g
NingXia Wolfberry Puree (Lycium barbarum), Blueberry Juice Concentrate (Vaccinium corymbosum), Plum Juice Concentrate (Prunus domestica), Cherry Juice Concentrate (Prunus avium), Aronia Juice Concentrate (Aronia melanocarpa), Pomegranate Juice Concentrate (Punica granatum)
Proprietary Essential Oil blend - 100 mg
Grape (Vitis vinifera) seed extract, Orange EO (Citrus sinensis), Yuzu EO (Citrus junos), Lemon EO (Citrus limon), Tangerine EO (Citrus reticulata)
Other ingredients - Tartaric acid, natural blueberry flavor, pure vanilla extract, malic acid, pectin, sodium benzoate/natural, stevia extract.

WHAT THE INGREDIENTS DO
- Calcium - for healthy bones, muscles, nervous system, and heart.
- Iron - supports healthy blood and immunity; may support fatigue.
- Sodium - supports nerve impulses and maintains the balance of water and minerals.

Proprietary NingXia Red® Blend
- NingXia Wolfberry Puree - rich in vitamins and minerals including Vitamins A and C along with Zinc and Iron. Unusually high in complex carbohydrates, this high antioxidant puree boosts the immune system and has been found to be particularly beneficial to support liver and eye health.
- Blueberry Juice Concentrate, Plum Juice Concentrate, Cherry Juice Concentrate, Aronia Juice Concentrate, Pomegranate Juice Concentrate - a unique collection of all extremely high antioxidant rich fruit juices that are known to boost immunity and protect against oxidative stress.

Proprietary Essential Oil blend - 100 mg
- Grapeseed extract - rich in antioxidants including flavonoids and phytonutrients; protects against oxidative stress and supports healthy whole-body wellness.
- Orange, Yuzu, Lemon, Tangerine - high in limonene, these antioxidant rich citrus oils boost immunity, cleanse toxins from the body, support circulation and digestive health and stimulate lymphatic drainage. Tangerine is particularly beneficial for respiratory health while Yuzu has beneficial properties that support nerve and brain health.

Other ingredients -
- Tartaric acid - antioxidant.
- Natural blueberry flavor - to enhance flavor.
- Pure vanilla extract - to enhance flavor.
- Malic acid - found in apples and pears; supports energy.
- Pectin - supports digestion and blood.
- Sodium benzoate (natural source) - natural preservative.
- Stevia extract - adds no-calorie sweetness.

COMMENTS FROM YOUNG LIVING

"Young Living NingXia Red® benefits include support for energy levels, normal cellular function, and whole-body and normal eye health. A daily shot of 2–4 ounces helps support overall wellness with powerful antioxidants. The wolfberries sourced for NingXia Red® hail from the NingXia province in northern China. This superfruit has one of the highest percentages of fiber of any whole food and contains zeaxanthin—a carotenoid important to maintaining healthy vision. It also contains polysaccharides, amino acids, and symbiotic vitamin mineral pairs that when present together promote optimum internal absorption. By using whole wolfberry puree—juice, peel, seeds, and fruit—Young Living is able to maintain more of the desired health-supporting benefits in every bottle of NingXia Red®."

DIRECTIONS FOR USE

- Drink 1-2 ounces twice daily. Best served chilled. Shake well before use. Refrigerate after opening and consume within 30 days. Do not drink directly from the bottle. Do not use if the seal is broken.
- Blend NingXia Red® into your smoothie, acai bowl, or morning juice as part of a quick, convenient breakfast.
- Chill and serve NingXia Red® to family and guests at gatherings and celebrations when you're looking for a healthy alternative to sparkling drinks.
- Treat children to this tasty drink instead of sugary sodas or juice cocktails.
- Combine with NingXia NITRO® for a nourishing drink that also supports cognitive wellness.
- Add a drop or two of your favorite dietary essential oil for an extra flavor boost! Try Peppermint, Thieves®, Cinnamon Bark, or Grapefruit.

The statements about the supplement and the ingredients have not been evaluated by the Food and Drug Administration. Young Living® products are not intended to diagnose, treat, cure, or prevent any disease.

NINGXIA NITRO®

NingXia NITRO® is a non-habit forming energy shot that contains natural sources of energy from green tea extract, ginseng, and choline to help support mental clarity. It should be used anytime there is a need for heightened cognition and energy. Consider using NITRO® for the afternoon lull, to support head tension, for added clarity before a test or presentation, for an energy boost before a workout, or anytime extra energy is needed.

INGREDIENTS
Calories per serving - 20
Carbohydrates 5 g (DV 2%)
Sugars 4 g
- Niacin (as niacinamide) - 10 mg (DV 50%)
- Vitamin B6 (as pyridoxine HCl) - 1 mg (DV 4%)
- Vitamin B12 (as methylcobalamin) - 6 µg (DV 100%)
- Iodine - 75 µg (DV 50%)

Proprietary NITRO® Energy blend – 476 mg
- D-Ribose
- Green tea extract
- Mulberry leaf extract
- Korean ginseng extract
- Choline (as Choline bitartrate)

Proprietary NITRO® Alert oil blend – 5 mg
- Vanilla absolute oil
- Chocolate oil
- Yerba mate oil
- Spearmint oil
- Peppermint oil
- Nutmeg oil
- Black Pepper oil
- Wolfberry seed oil

NITRO® juice blend concentrate - Cherry, Kiwi, Blueberry, Acerola, Bilberry, Black currant, Raspberry, Strawberry, Cranberry, Coconut nectar, Natural flavors, Pectin, Xanthan gum
Other Ingredients - Purified water
NOTE: Contains dairy and tree nut (coconut)

WHAT THE INGREDIENTS DO
- Niacin B3 - converts food into usable energy.
- Vitamin B6 - supports healthy nerves, skin, and red blood cells.
- Vitamin B12 - supports red blood cells, brain health, eye health, skin health, DNA production, cardiovascular support, and converts the food you eat into energy.
- Iodine - supports the thyroid, metabolic rate, maintains energy levels, promotes removal of toxins, boosts immunity and is critical in the prevention of enlarged thyroid gland.

Proprietary NITRO® Energy blend – 476mg
- D-Ribose - supports energy; supports heart metabolism and improved muscle function.
- Green tea extract - antioxidants that support energy, heart, liver and brain health.
- Mulberry leaf extract - antioxidant to support cholesterol, triglycerides, and glucose.
- Korean ginseng extract - improves antioxidant activity in cells and mental fatigue.
- Choline (as Choline bitartrate) - cognitive enhancer that supports brain health.

Proprietary NITRO® Alert oil blend – 5mg
- Vanilla absolute oil - flavor enhancer and may reduce stress and peace.
- Chocolate oil - (absolute) may relax muscles and help balance the body and the mind.
- Yerba mate oil - antioxidants support energy, immunity, and clarity.
- Spearmint oil - soothes digestion, cools and promotes energy and emotionally uplifting.
- Peppermint oil - supports digestion, brain function, immunity, energy, and focus.
- Nutmeg oil - supports lymphatic, immune, and digestive health. Supports adrenals.
- Black Pepper oil - supports the liver; helps promote bioavailability of other supplements.
- Wolfberry seed oil - exceptionally high in essential fatty acids; stimulates intracellular oxygenation and blood circulation.

NITRO® juice blend concentrate -
- Cherry - antioxidants to support immunity and protect against oxidative stress.
- Kiwi - antioxidants with vitamin C, vitamin K, vitamin E, folate, and potassium.
- Bilberry - supports blood vessels, cellular health, and circulation.
- Acerola - high in vitamin C, supports immune health.
- Bilberry - strengthens blood vessels, improves circulation.
- Black currant - antioxidants with vitamin C for immunity.
- Raspberry - antioxidants with vitamins and minerals.
- Strawberry - improves the skin and supports a healthy immune system.
- Cranberry - supports renal system, immunity, and blood.
- Coconut nectar - contains a wide range of vitamins, minerals, and amino acids.
- Natural flavors - extracted from fruit or fruit juice to enhance flavor.
- Pectin - supports digestion and blood.
- Xanthan gum - adds sweet taste.

COMMENTS FROM YOUNG LIVING

"When you need a midday boost, it's easy to reach for things like soda and energy drinks. Skip the sugary solution and reboot with an option from Young Living. With NingXia NITRO®, you'll get a quick pick-me-up without the sugar or caffeine overload. Infused with essential oils, botanical extracts, D-ribose, Korean ginseng, and green tea extract, NingXia NITRO® supports alertness, as well as cognitive and physical fitness. A great support for body and mind wellness, use NingXia NITRO® for running, weight-lifting, or getting through your afternoon slump. The naturally occurring caffeine in Young Living's NingXia NITRO® supports normal energy levels and alertness to help you with a busy day or a tough workout. Stash NITRO® wherever you need it! The small, convenient packaging makes it a great addition to your office desk, gym bag, or purse. Each box contains 14 20ml tubes."

DIRECTIONS FOR USE

Consume NingXia NITRO® directly from the tube or mix with 1 oz. of NingXia Red® or 4 oz. of water to enhance physical performance, clear the mind, or anytime you need a pick-me-up. Best served chilled. Shake well before using and refrigerate after opening.

The statements about the supplement and the ingredients have not been evaluated by the Food and Drug Administration. Young Living® products are not intended to diagnose, treat, cure, or prevent any disease.

NINGXIA ZYNG™

Forget those really-bad-for-you energy drinks and sodas! NingXia Zyng™ is the healthy alternative. Drink Zyng™ when you need a quick pick-me-up, or enjoy a NingXia "cocktail" by combining a can of NingXia Zyng™, 2 ounces of NingXia Red®, and one tube of NingXia NITRO® with 3 drops Lime Vitality™, 3 drops Tangerine Vitality™, and 1 drop Peppermint Vitality™.

INGREDIENTS

Calories per serving 35
Total Carbohydrates 9 g
Sugars 8 g
- Vitamin A - (DV 10%)
- Vitamin B6 - (DV 50%)
- Vitamin E - (DV 10%)
- Niacin - (DV 50%)
- Pantothenic acid - (DV 50%)
- Carbonated water
- Evaporated cane sugar
- Pear juice concentrate
- Wolfberry (Lycium barbarum) puree
- Citric acid
- Blackberry juice concentrate
- Natural flavor
- White tea leaf extract
- Stevia rebaudiana leaf extract
- D-calcium pantothenate
- Niacinamide
- Black Pepper (Piper nigrum) fruit oil
- Lime (Citrus latifolia) peel oil
- D-alpha-tocopherol acetate
- Pyridoxine hydrochloride
- Retinyl palmitate

WHAT THE INGREDIENTS DO
- Carbonated water - makes the drink bubbly and sometimes more enjoyable to consume.
- Evaporated cane sugar - less-processed, more nutritious form of cane sugar.
- Pear juice concentrate - antioxidants with vitamin C, K, B, potassium, copper, phosphorus, magnesium, calcium, and iron, as well as others.
- Wolfberry puree - supports immunity, as well as healthy regeneration of tissues and cells.
- Citric acid - preservative and flavor enhancer; antioxidant and alkalizing properties.
- Blackberry juice concentrate - antioxidant with manganese, copper, Vitamins A, C, E and K.
- Natural flavor - extracted from fruit or fruit juice to enhance flavor.
- White tea leaf extract - high amount of antioxidants; protects cells from free radicals.
- Stevia rebaudiana leaf extract - healthy, no calorie natural sweetener.
- D-calcium pantothenate - antioxidants to reduce the amount of water lost through the skin.
- Niacinamide (B3) - converts consumed food into usable energy.
- Black Pepper fruit oil - supports liver and energy; helps bioavailability of supplements.
- Lime peel oil - supports digestion and is a natural detoxifier.
- D-alpha-tocopherol acetate - Vitamin E that exhibits the greatest bioavailability in the body.
- Pyridoxine hydrochloride (B6) - supports the health of nerves, skin, and red blood cells.
- Retinyl palmitate - used as an antioxidant, a source of Vitamin A in a more stable form.

COMMENTS FROM YOUNG LIVING
"A hydrating splash of essential oil-infused goodness, NingXia Zyng™ uses the same whole-fruit wolfberry puree found in our popular superfruit supplement, NingXia Red®. We add sparkling water, pear and blackberry juices, and a hint of Lime and Black Pepper essential oils for a dynamic, unique taste. You'll enjoy a refreshing boost that's full of flavor without artificial flavors and preservatives. With natural flavors and sweeteners, white tea extract, and added vitamins, NingXia Zyng™ delivers 35 mg of naturally occurring caffeine and only 35 calories per can, making it a sweet, guilt-free boost for your early morning, long afternoon, or anytime you need a little Zyng!"

DIRECTIONS FOR USE
Drink 1 can as desired. Best served chilled. Lightly invert can before opening.
CAUTIONS: Contains naturally occurring caffeine from white tea extract (35 mg), so use in moderation if consuming after 3 p.m. Not intended for young children or those who may be sensitive to caffeine.

The statements about the supplement and the ingredients have not been evaluated by the Food and Drug Administration. Young Living® products are not intended to diagnose, treat, cure, or prevent any disease.

OMEGAGIZE3™

There are so many fish oil omega-3 fatty acid supplements from which to choose, but Young Living® has far exceeded all the others with OmegaGize3™! OmegaGize3™ is a core omega-3 supplement infused with an essential oil blend. Many of the Young Living® supplements are infused with essential oils. Essential oils, when taken internally, can support health in a myriad of ways. Studies have shown that when infused with essential oils, the nutrients in the supplements become more bioavailable.

INGREDIENTS
Calories per serving - 10
Total fat - 1 g (DV 1%)
Vitamin D (as cholecalciferol) - 24 mcg (DV 120%)
Proprietary OmegaGize3™ Blend – 1.1 g
- Omega-3 fatty acids (from Basa fish oil) - 445 mg
- Eicosapentaenoic acid (EPA) - 135 mg
- Docosahexaenoic acid (DHA) - 310 mg
- Coenzyme Q10 (as ubiquinone)

Omega Enhancement Blend – 156 mg
- Clove flower bud oil (Syzygium aromaticum)
- German Chamomile flower oil (Matricaria recutita)
- Spearmint leaf oil (Mentha spicata)

Other ingredients - Gelatin, Rice bran oil, Silicon dioxide, Purified water, Mixed carotenoids
Contains fish (Basa)

WHAT THE INGREDIENTS DO
- Vitamin D (D3) - supports healthy bones and helps support immunity. Helps boost weight loss, and improves moods.

Proprietary OmegaGize3™ Blend
- Omega-3 fatty acids - supports healthy brain and cardiovascular health.
- Eicosapentaenoic acid (EPA) - supports the heart and menopause symptoms.
- Docosahexaenoic acid (DHA) - supports the brain and fetal development.
- Coenzyme Q10 - helps produce energy, normal growth, maintenance and repair.

Omega Enhancement Blend
- Clove flower bud oil - supports a healthy microbial balance in the body.
- German Chamomile flower oil - for stomach upset, and helps minimize flatulence.
- Spearmint leaf oil - Soothes digestion and promotes energy.

Other ingredients - Gelatin, Rice bran oil, Silicon dioxide, Purified water, Mixed carotenoids - capsule and substrates.

COMMENTS FROM YOUNG LIVING
"OmegaGize3™ combines the power of three core daily supplements - omega 3 fatty acids, vitamin D-3, and CoQ10 (ubiquinone). These supplements combine with our proprietary enhancement essential oil blend to create an omega-3, DHA-rich fish oil supplement that may support general wellness. Used daily these ingredients work synergistically to support normal brain, heart, eye, and joint health."

DIRECTIONS FOR USE
Take 4 liquid ocean capsules daily, 2 in the morning and 2 in the evening for daily maintenance. Take eight capsules for greater health benefits.

The statements about the supplement and the ingredients have not been evaluated by the Food and Drug Administration. Young Living® products are not intended to diagnose, treat, cure, or prevent any disease.

PD 80/20™

PD 80/20™ is the most basic of all the hormone supplements but has a perfect balance of pregnenolone to natural DHEA from wild yams. This supplement contains 400 mg of pregnenolone and 100 mg of DHEA which is where its name is derived from - 80% Pregnenolone to 20% DHEA.

INGREDIENTS
- Pregnenolone 400 mg
- DHEA (dehydroepiandrosterone) derived from wild yams 100 mg

Other ingredients - Rice flour, gelatin (for capsule)

WHAT THE INGREDIENTS DO
- Pregnenolone - a precursor hormone that increases the production of all hormones in the body such as progesterone, estrogen, and cortisol. It supports fatigue, increases energy, supports memory, supports motivation, helps increase libido, and may help improve mood swings. According to a study published in 2009 by Marx, Keefe, and Buchanan, in Neuropsychopharmacology titled "Proof-of-concept trial with the neurosteroid pregnenolone targeting cognitive and negative symptoms in schizophrenia," they found that patients with schizophrenia saw improvements with their symptoms when they used pregnenolone for eight weeks.
- DHEA (dehydroepiandrosterone) - a precursor hormone that helps with cognition, healthy emotions, libido, and muscle and bone mass. It may also help with vaginal dryness.

Other ingredients
- Rice flour - substrate powder.
- Gelatin - capsule (from animals). Vegetarians can open the capsule and put into a drink.

NOTE: there are no essential oils in this supplement.

COMMENTS FROM YOUNG LIVING
"PD 80/20™ is a dietary supplement formulated to help maximize internal health and support the endocrine system. It contains pregnenolone and DHEA, two substances produced naturally by the body that decline with age. Pregnenolone is the key precursor for the body's production of estrogen, DHEA, and progesterone, and it also has an impact on mental acuity and memory. DHEA is involved in maintaining the health of the cardiovascular and immune systems."

DIRECTIONS FOR USE
Start with 1 capsule per day, then increase to 2 capsules per day as needed.

The statements about the supplement and the ingredients have not been evaluated by the Food and Drug Administration. Young Living® products are not intended to diagnose, treat, cure, or prevent any disease.

PARAFREE™

ParaFree™ supports digestion, circulation, respiratory, and immunity by focusing on helping your body rid itself of unwanted hitch-hikers. This essential oil capsule combines powerful essential oils that cleanse the body and support oxidative stress. Many parasites can be found in the human body. We have almost 300 species of parasitic worms that we could contract over our lifetime.

INGREDIENTS

ParaFree™ Blend - 2250 mg

- Sesame (Sesamum indicum) seed oil
- Cumin (Cuminum cyminum) seed oil
- Olive (Olea europaea) fruit oil
- Anise (Pimpinella anisum) fruit oil
- Fennel (Foeniculum vulgare) seed oil
- Vetiver (Vetiveria zizanioides) root oil
- Bay Laurel (Laurus nobilis) leaf oil
- Nutmeg (Myristica fragrans) seed oil
- Tea tree (Melaleuca alternifolia) leaf oil
- Thyme (Thymus vulgaris) leaf oil
- Clove (syzygium aromaticum) flower bud oil
- Ocotea (Ocotea quixos) leaf oil
- Dorado Azul (Hyptis suaveolens) aerial parts oil
- Tarragon (Artemisia dracunculus) leaf oil
- Ginger (Zingiber offiicinale) root oil
- Peppermint (Mentha piperita) aerial parts oil
- Juniper (Juniperus osteosperma) aerial parts oil
- Lemongrass (Cymbopogon flexuosus) leaf oil
- Patchouli (Pogostemon cablin) leaf oil

Other Ingredients -
Fish gelatin (tilapia or carp for capsule), Glycerin, Water

WHAT THE INGREDIENTS DO

ParaFree™ Blend

- Sesame seed oil - carrier oil rich in Vitamin B with high antioxidant properties.
- Cumin seed oil - aids in digestion and promotes a reduction of potential flatulence.
- Olive fruit oil - antioxidants protect cells and promote cardiovascular health.
- Anise fruit oil - helps keep blood sugar levels stable, improves digestion.
- Fennel seed oil - improves digestion, and is a mild appetite suppressant.
- Vetiver root oil - known for its soothing, grounding abilities.
- Bay Laurel leaf oil - is renewing and purifying.
- Nutmeg seed oil - supports lymphatic, digestive, and immune health; promotes energy.
- Tea tree leaf oil - supports respiratory and intestinal tract. Research: may help prevent antibiotic resistance; positive synergistic effect when combined with antibiotics.
- Thyme leaf oil - supports digestive cleansing, urinary, immune, and respiratory systems.
- Clove flower bud oil - antioxidants support a healthy microbial balance in the body.
- Ocotea leaf oil - stimulates digestion and supports the liver; supports blood sugar, cardiovascular, and blood flow; helps curb cravings and promote feelings of fullness.
- Dorado Azul oil - supports the respiratory system.
- Tarragon leaf oil - improves digestion, fights bacteria.
- Ginger root oil - supports digestion, cleanses bowels, minimizes flatulence.
- Peppermint oil - supports digestion, brain function, immunity, energy, and focus.
- Juniper oil - is a powerful cleanser and detoxifier.
- Lemongrass leaf oil - supports immunity, digestion, can help lower cholesterol levels.
- Patchouli leaf oil - is soothing and releasing to the body.

COMMENTS FROM YOUNG LIVING

"ParaFree™ is formulated with an advanced blend of some of the strongest essential oils studied for their cleansing abilities. This formula also includes the added benefits of sesame seed oil and olive oil."

DIRECTIONS FOR USE

Take 3 softgels twice daily or as needed. For best results, take for 21 days and rest for seven days. Cycle may be repeated three times. Take on an empty stomach for maximum results.

The statements about the supplement and the ingredients have not been evaluated by the Food and Drug Administration. Young Living® products are not intended to diagnose, treat, cure, or prevent any disease.

POWERGIZE™

A favorite among athletes, Powergize™ can be utilized by any adult wishing to boost their physical game. Formulated with Ashwagandha root (also found in EndoGize™), PowerGize™ helps support male testosterone, physical performance, and sexual drive. Both men and women may use this supplement.

INGREDIENTS
- Vitamin B6 (as pyridoxine HCL)12 mg
- Magnesium (as magnesium bisglycinate) 20 mg
- Zinc (as zinc glycinate chelate) 5 mg

PowerGize™ Energy Blend 995.25 mg
- Ashwagandha (Withania somnifera) root extract
- Longjack (Eurycoma longifolia) root powder
- Fenugreek (Trigonella foenum-graecum) (50% saponin) seed extract
- Epimedium (Epimedium brevicornum) leaf powder
- Desert hyacinth (Cistanche tubulosa) root powder
- Tribulus (Tribulus Terrestris) (45% saponin) fruit/leaf extract
- Muira puama (Ptychopetalum olacoides) bark powder

Essential Oils - Idaho Blue spruce (Picea pungens) aerial parts oil, Goldenrod (Solidago canadensis) flowering top oil, Cassia (Cinnamomum aromaticum) branch/leaf oil

Other ingredients - Hypromellose, Rice flour, Silicon dioxide

WHAT THE INGREDIENTS DO
- Vitamin B6 - supports brain development, nervous system, and immune system.
- Magnesium - aids in normal function of the cells, nerves, muscles, bones, and heart.
- Zinc - supports immune function, tissue growth, and skin, eye and heart health.

PowerGize™ Energy Blend
- Ashwagandha root extract - supports immunity, mental clarity, concentration, and alertness. May improve memory and brain function, may help reduce cortisol levels when chronically stressed, and supports healthy emotions, peace, and stress.
- Longjack root powder - may boost testosterone, increase energy, and physical endurance.
- Fenugreek seed extract - supports digestion and blood; improves exercise performance.
- Epimedium leaf powder - boosts stamina, focus, and energy.
- Desert hyacinth root powder - supports cardiovascular and renal health; muscle building.
- Tribulus fruit/leaf extract - enhances libido, natural diuretic properties, supports heart.
- Muira puama bark powder - promotes nerve function and cognitive health.
- Idaho Blue spruce aerial parts oil - supports respiratory, endocrine, and immune health.
- Goldenrod flowering top oil - supports respiratory, lymphatic, circulatory and heart health.
- Cassia branch/leaf oil - supports nervous, digestive, circulatory and immune systems.

Other ingredients
- Hypromellose, Rice flour, Silicon dioxide - capsule and substrate.

COMMENTS FROM YOUNG LIVING
"Inspire your inner athlete with PowerGize™! This supplement is specially formulated to help individuals of all ages boost stamina and performance. PowerGize™ helps sustain energy levels, strength, mental and physical vibrancy, and vitality when used in addition to physical activity. PowerGize™ is also formulated with KSM-66, a premium ashwagandha root extract, which is touted for its properties that support immunity, mental clarity, concentration, and alertness."

DIRECTIONS FOR USE
Take 2 capsules daily.

The statements about the supplement and the ingredients have not been evaluated by the Food and Drug Administration. Young Living® products are not intended to diagnose, treat, cure, or prevent any disease.

PROSTATE HEALTH™

Specifically formulated for men, Prostate Health™ targets key elements to support the prostate. It helps elevate moods, balances testosterone levels, supports the body's inflammatory response, and provides antioxidant support. The essential oils in Prostate Health™ are known to help support healthy digestion.

INGREDIENTS
- Saw palmetto (Serenoa Replens/serrulata) fruit extract
- Pumpkin (cucurbita pepo) seed oil
- Geranium (Pelargonium graveolens) flower/leaf oil
- Fennel (foeniculum vulare) seed oil
- Lavender (Lavandula angustifolia) flowering top oil
- Myrtle (Myrtus communis) leaf oil
- Peppermint (Mentha piperita) aerial parts oil

Other ingredients - porcine gelatin, water, silica

WHAT THE INGREDIENTS DO
- Saw palmetto fruit extract - balances testosterone and improves prostate health.
- Pumpkin seed oil - reduces inflammation, supports a healthy prostate; supports mental health and combats stress and supports healthy emotions.
- Geranium flower/leaf oil - promotes urination, reduces inflammation, balances hormones.
- Fennel seed oil - improves digestion, and is a mild appetite suppressant.
- Lavender flowering top oil - supports moods, immunity, and respiratory systems.
- Myrtle leaf oil - supports urinary tract, bladder, digestion, and respiratory health.
- Peppermint oil - supports digestion, brain function, immunity, energy, and focus.

Other ingredients
- Porcine gelatin, Water, and Silica - capsule and substrate.

COMMENTS FROM YOUNG LIVING
"Prostate Health™ is uniquely formulated for men concerned with supporting the male glandular system and maintaining healthy, normal prostate function. Prostate Health™ is an essential oil supplement featuring powerful saw palmetto and pumpkin seed oil—ingredients known for their support of a healthy prostate gland. A proprietary blend of pure Geranium, Fennel, Myrtle, Lavender, and Peppermint essential oils provides the body with key components. The benefits of liquid capsules include a targeted release for ideal absorption and minimal aftertaste. For maximum benefit, Prostate Health™ should be taken consistently over time."

DIRECTIONS FOR USE
Take 1 liquid capsule twice daily.

The statements about the supplement and the ingredients have not been evaluated by the Food and Drug Administration. Young Living® products are not intended to diagnose, treat, cure, or prevent any disease.

PURE PROTEIN™ COMPLETE

Pure Protein™ Complete shake mix comes in both vanilla and chocolate. This shake will keep you full much longer than other meal replacement shakes. This is because it contains five different proteins that your body processes at different rates. Pure Protein™ Complete is gluten free. It helps you have sustained energy and contains digestive enzymes and amino acids that are crucial for energy production and healthy immune function.

INGREDIENTS
Calories - 170
Calories from Fat - 20
Total Fat - 2.5 g (DV 4%)
Saturated Fat - 1.5 g (DV 8%)
Trans Fat - 0 g
Cholesterol - 50 mg (DV 17%)
Sodium - 240 mg (DV 10%)
Total Carbohydrate - 14 g (DV 5%)
Dietary Fiber - 2 g (DV 8%)
Sugars - 9 g
Protein - 25 g (DV 50%)
- Thiamin (as thiamin hydrochloride) 0.75 mg (DV 50%)
- Riboflavin 8.85 mg (DV 50%)
- Niacin 10 mg (DV 50%)
- Vitamin B6 (as pyridoxine hydrochloride) 1mg (DV 50%
- Vitamin B12 (as methylcobalamin) 3 mcg (DV 50%)
- Biotin 150 mcg (DV 50%)
- Pantothenic Acid (as d-calcium pantothenate) 5 mg (DV 50%)
- Calcium - (as d-calcium pantothenate) 100 mg (DV 10%)
- Zinc (as zinc picolinate) 15 mg (DV 100%)

Pure Protein™ Proprietary Blend - 31.75 gm
- rBGH-free whey protein concentrate
- Pea protein isolate
- Goat whey protein concentrate
- Egg albumin
- Organic hemp seed protein
- Ancient peat
- Apple extract

Enzyme Proprietary Complex - 55 gm
- Amylase, Protease, Lipase, Cellulase, Lactase & L. acidophilus, Papain, Bromelain

Amino Acid Blend - L-leucine, L-isoleucine, L-valine, L-methionine, L-lysine, L-glutamine
- Sodium chloride
- Stevia (Stevia rebaudiana)
- Orange (Citrus sinensis) rind oil
- Luo han guo (Siraitia grosvenorii) fruit extract

Other Ingredients - Cane Sugar, Cocoa Powder, Natural flavors, Xanthan gum

WHAT THE INGREDIENTS DO
- Thiamin (B1) - beneficial to a healthy nervous system.
- Riboflavin (B2) - needed for overall growth. It also helps support energy levels.
- Niacin (B3) - helps lower cholesterol, ease arthritis and boost brain function.
- Vitamin B6 - supports the health of nerves, skin, and red blood cells.
- Vitamin B12 - supports the body to make red blood cells.
- Biotin (B7) - supports a healthy metabolism and creates enzymes.

- Pantothenic Acid (B5) - reduces the amount of water lost through the skin.
- Calcium - specific calcium to reduce the amount of water lost through the skin.
- Zinc - supports inflammation, blood, and heart.

Pure Protein™ Proprietary Blend -
- rBGH-free whey protein concentrate - stimulates muscle growth.
- Pea protein isolate - easily digested protein.
- Goat whey protein concentrate - promotes a healthy immune and digestive system.
- Egg albumin - excellent source of protein.
- Organic hemp seed protein - easily digestible, plant-based complete protein.
- Ancient peat and Apple extract (as elevATP) - supports ATP production for energy.

Enzyme Proprietary Complex -
- Alpha and Beta amylase - breaks down starch, breads, and pasta.
- Protease - digests proteins to allow absorption of amino acids; converts food to energy.
- Lipase - breaks down dietary fats and oils. Helps liver function.
- Cellulase - breaks down man-made fiber, plant fiber, fruits, and veggies.
- Lactase & L. acidophilus - breaks down dairy sugars and help minimize lactose intolerance.
- Papain - digestive aid, may help parasites, shingles, diarrhea, and runny nose.
- Bromelain - breaks down peptides and amino acids; supports inflammation in the blood.

Amino acid blend -
- L-leucine, L-isoleucine & L-valine - supports the brain, liver, and fatigue during exercise.
- L-methionine - supports growth of new blood vessels; supports the immune system.
- L-lysine - converts fatty acids into energy; supports absorption of calcium; supports stress.
- L-glutamine - boosts immune cell activity in the gut; supports infection and inflammation.

Other Ingredients -
- Sodium chloride - supports fluid balance and electrolytes.
- Stevia - no calorie natural sweetener.
- Orange rind oil - supports immunity and improves blood flow.
- Luo han guo fruit extract - adds sweetness with no calories (Monk fruit).
- Cane Sugar - natural sweetener.
- Cocoa Powder - natural flavor (chocolate flavor only).
- Natural flavors - extracted from fruit or fruit juice to enhance flavor.
- Xanthan gum - adds sweet taste.

Allergens: Contains dairy and egg derived ingredients.

COMMENTS FROM YOUNG LIVING

"Pure Protein™ Complete is a comprehensive protein supplement that combines a proprietary 5-Protein Blend, amino acids, and ancient peat and apple extract to deliver 25 grams of protein per serving in two delicious flavors, Vanilla Spice and Chocolate Deluxe. Its foundation of cow and goat whey, pea protein, egg white protein, and organic hemp seed protein provide a full range of amino acids including - D-aspartic acid, Threonine, L-serine, Glutamic acid, Glycine, Alanine, Valine, Methionine, Isoleucine, Leucine, Tyrosine, Phenylalanine, Lysine, Histidine, Arginine, Proline, Hydroxyproline, Cystine, Tryptophan, and Cysteine. Along with a proprietary enzyme blend, these amino acids support overall protein utilization in the body. Ancient peat and apple extract, along with a powerful B-vitamin blend, complete the formula. Together they support ATP production, the energy currency of the body. This innovative formula makes Pure Protein™ Complete the perfect option for those looking for a high protein supplement that features a full range of amino acids."

DIRECTIONS FOR USE

Add 2 scoops of Pure Protein™ Complete to 8 oz. of cold water. May also be mixed with rice, almond, or other milk. Shake or stir until smooth. For added flavor, add fruit or essential oils. Blend with ice for a nice shake.

The statements about the supplement and the ingredients have not been evaluated by the Food and Drug Administration. Young Living® products are not intended to diagnose, treat, cure, or prevent any disease.

REHEMOGEN™

Rehemogen™ helps cleanse your intestinal tract as a mild laxative and supports healthy blood and detoxification. It helps to calm nervous energy and supports the digestive, nervous, renal, respiratory, lymphatic, endocrine, and immune systems. Rehemogen™ is a tincture, which means it is in liquid form that you may add from the dropper bottle directly to water or juice. You may also put each half dropper into a veggie capsule. Three veggie capsules will hold one serving.

INGREDIENTS
- Red clover (Trifolium pratense) blossom
- Licorice (Glycyrrhiza glabra) root
- Poke (Phytolacca americana) root
- Peach (Prunus persica) bark
- Oregon grape (Berberis aquifolium) root
- Stillingia (S. sylvatica) root
- Sarsaparilla (Smilax medica) root
- Cascara sagrada (Frangula purshiana) bark
- Prickly ash (Zanthoxylum americanum) bark
- Burdock (Arctium lappa) root
- Buckthorn (Rhamnus frangula) bark
- Roman chamomile (Chamaemelum nobile) flower oil
- Rosemary (Rosmarinus officinalis) leaf oil
- Thyme (Thymus vulgaris) leaf oil
- Tea tree (Melaleuca alternifolia) leaf oil

Other ingredients - Distilled water, Ethanol

WHAT THE INGREDIENTS DO
- Red clover blossom - source of vitamin A, B-complex, C, F and P, and trace minerals.
- Licorice root - mild laxative; softens, lubricates, and nourishes the intestinal tract.
- Poke root - stimulates congested and sluggish glandular system.
- Peach bark - strengthens the nervous system and stimulates the flow of urine.
- Oregon grape root - supports immunity, diarrhea, and digestion.
- Stillingia root - effective glandular stimulant as well as an activator for the liver.
- Sarsaparilla root - hormone balancing; supports metabolism.
- Cascara sagrada bark - moves waste out of the body. NOTE - Turns stool black.
- Prickly ash bark - supports circulation; improves blood purification.
- Burdock root - supports kidneys, lymphatics, and increases the flow of urine.
- Buckthorn bark - supports the gastrointestinal tract; eases constipation.
- Royal jelly - produced by honey bees. Source of B vitamins. Supports the cardiovascular, kidneys, lungs, and immune systems.
- Roman chamomile flower oil - antioxidant; supports GI tract by reducing digestive discomfort.
- Rosemary leaf oil - aids in digestion and supports liver cleansing.
- Thyme leaf oil - supports digestive cleansing, promotes healthy renal and urinary systems.
- Tea tree leaf oil - supports respiratory and intestinal tract.

Other ingredients - Distilled water and Ethanol - tincture base.

COMMENTS FROM YOUNG LIVING
"Rehemogen™ contains Cascara sagrada, red clover, poke root, prickly ash bark, and burdock root, which have been historically used for their cleansing and building properties. Rehemogen™ is also formulated with essential oils to enhance digestion."

DIRECTIONS FOR USE
Take 3 half droppers (3ml) 3 times daily in distilled water just prior to or with meals containing protein. Shake well before using. Refrigerate after opening.
Do not exceed recommended dosage. Not for long term use.

SLEEPESSENCE™

SleepEssence™ is an essential oil filled capsule used to support natural sleep patterns to help calm your mind so you can fall asleep faster. It contains a small amount of melatonin to help you drift off to sleep and the oils, when taken consistently over time, help you stay asleep longer. You may take 1 capsule for light support or 2 if you need more help getting a restful night's sleep.

INGREDIENTS

SleepEssence™ Blend -
Contains 12.8 drops total of Coconut carrier and pure essential oils
- Lavender (Lavandula officinalis) flowering top oil
- Vetiver (Vetiveria zizanioides) root oil
- Valerian (Valeriana officinalis) root oil
- Tangerine (Citrus reticulata) rind oil
- Rue (Ruta graveolens) flower oil
- Melatonin 3.2 mg per serving (2 capsules)

Other Ingredients - Lecithin, Coconut (Cocos nucifera) fruit oil, Carrageenan, Glycerin, Modified cornstarch, Sorbitol, Water
NOTE: Contains tree nuts (Coconut)

WHAT THE INGREDIENTS DO
- Lavender oil - provides antioxidant protection; supports moods and sleep.
- Vetiver oil - antioxidant; supports insomnia and stress. Promotes relaxation and calm.
- Valerian oil - supports asleep, calms moods, reduces brain activity, improves sleep quality, and relaxes muscles.
- Tangerine oil - relaxes nerves and muscles, reduces tension, promotes healthy sleep.
- Rue oil - antioxidant; relaxing benefits.
- Melatonin - improves sleep quality. Helps people with disrupted circadian rhythm. Leads to the recovery of pituitary and thyroid functions. Has anti-inflammatory and antioxidant effects. Strengthens the immune system. Helps to relieve stress.

Other Ingredients -
- Lecithin - supports positive moods and peace.
- Coconut fruit oil - carrier base.
- Carrageenan - supports immunity, antioxidant, and prebiotic.
- Glycerin - adds base and sweet taste.
- Modified cornstarch - stabilizer and emulsifier for ingredients.
- Sorbitol - sweetener and mild laxative.
- Water - supplement base.

COMMENTS FROM YOUNG LIVING
"SleepEssence™ contains four powerful Young Living Therapeutic Grade™ essential oils that have unique sleep-enhancing properties in a softgel vegetarian capsule for easy ingestion. Combining Lavender, Vetiver, Valerian, and Ruta Graveolens essential oils with the hormone melatonin—a well-known sleep aid—SleepEssence™ is a natural way to enable a full night's rest."

DIRECTIONS FOR USE
Take 1–2 softgels 30–60 minutes before bedtime.
CAUTION: Do not operate heavy machinery for 8-10 hours after using. Not recommended for long-term use or with products containing echinacea. Adult use only.

The statements about the supplement and the ingredients have not been evaluated by the Food and Drug Administration. Young Living® products are not intended to diagnose, treat, cure, or prevent any disease.

SLIQUE® PRODUCT LINE

Slique® products are designed to help you maintain a healthy weight. The Slique® system combines a meal replacement shake, snack bars, tea, gum and other items to help you reach your goals! This is a proven system and I highly recommend it!

SLIQUE® SHAKE

INGREDIENTS

Vitamin A	8%	Vitamin B12	6%
Vitamin C	20%	Biotin	8%
Calcium	2%	Pantothenic acid	10%
Iron	30%	Phosphorus	25%
Vitamin D	0%	Iodine	25%
Vitamin E	0%	Magnesium	20%
Thiamin	20%	Zinc	20%
Riboflavin	25%	Selenium	25%
Niacin	30%	Copper	25%
Vitamin B6	20%	Manganese	150%
Folate	15%	Chromium	10%

Ingredients List - Pea protein isolate, Isomalto-oligosaccharide, Medium chain triglycerides, Tapioca dextrose, Organic palm sugar, Natural flavor, Organic quinoa powder, Organic pumpkin seed protein, Xanthan gum, Strawberry fruit powder, Sodium citrate, Malic acid, Fruit & vegetable extract blend (Green tea leaf extract, Guarana seed extract, Red & white grape extracts, Grapefruit extract, Black carrot extract, Vitamin B3), Alfalfa grass juice powder, Organic wolfberry fruit powder, Stevia, Slique® essential oil (Grapefruit rind oil, Tangerine rind oil, Spearmint leaf oil, Lemon rind oil, Ocotea leaf oil, Stevia leaf extract), Vitamins and Minerals - Dipotassium phosphate, Monosodium phosphate, Magnesium oxide, Zinc gluconate, Organic B vitamin blend (Guava extract, Holy basil extract, Citrus limon extract), Ascorbic acid, Molybdenum glycinate, Niacin, Copper gluconate, Biotin, Vitamin A acetate, Sodium selenite, d-Calcium pantothenate, Chromium nicotinate glycinate chelate, Riboflavin, Pyridoxine HCl, Potassium iodide, Methylcobalamin

WHAT THE INGREDIENTS DO

- Pea protein isolate - is easily digested, rich in iron, arginine and branched-chain amino acids known to support muscle growth, feelings of fullness and cardiovascular health.
- Isomalto-oligosaccharide - (IMO) is a moderately sweet carbohydrate that occurs naturally in honey. It is also found in fermented foods and made up of carbohydrate chains that are resistant to digestion and low in calories.
- Medium chain triglycerides - (MCT) are fats found in foods like coconut oil. They are metabolized differently than long-chain triglycerides (LCT). MCTs include caproic acid (C6), caprylic acid (C8), capric acid (C10) and lauric acid (C12). Due to their shorter chain length, medium-chain triglycerides are more rapidly broken down and absorbed into the body. This makes them a fast energy source and less likely to be stored as fat.
- Tapioca dextrose - is a very quickly digested, simple sugar that offers immediate energy and is easily digested.
- Organic palm sugar - is the dehydrated sap of the coconut palm. It retains nutrient minerals like iron, zinc, calcium and potassium, along with some short-chain fatty acids like polyphenols and antioxidants.
- Natural flavor - is the flavorful constituents derived from a spice, fruit, vegetable, herbs, bark, bud, root, leaf or similar plant material.

- Organic quinoa powder - provides a complete plant-based protein whose benefits include improved solubility and stability. It contains all nine essential amino acids, is rich in omega 3, 6 & 9, potassium, iron, magnesium, and antioxidants. Naturally gluten-free, organic quinoa powder is easily digested and optimally absorbed because of its unique breakdown of starch bonds.
- Organic pumpkin seed protein - is a great source of tryptophan, manganese, magnesium, phosphorus, copper, protein, zinc and iron. Organic pumpkin seed protein can support normal blood pressure and sugar levels, as well as a healthy heart, bones, muscle and nerve function. Pumpkin seeds are full of antioxidants that may help reduce inflammation and support the immune system.
- Xanthan gum - is a complex exopolysaccharide, a polymer composed of sugar residues, secreted by a microorganism into the environment. Produced by plant-pathogenic bacterium – xanthan gum is often used as a thickening and stabilizing agent.
- Strawberry fruit powder - rich in fiber and helps the body to absorb key nutrients. Can help stabilize blood sugar levels and is high in vitamin C while low in calories.
- Sodium citrate - used as a food preservative, flavoring agent, and stabilizer.
- Malic acid - is a component of most fruits and can promote energy production, increase endurance and help prevent muscle fatigue while exercising; natural preservative.

Fruit & vegetable extract blend -
- Green tea leaf extract - is rich in antioxidants called catechins, which have been shown to increase antioxidant capacity and protect against oxidative stress.
- Guarana seed extract - contains the stimulants caffeine, theophylline and theobromine. It is also rich in antioxidants, including tannins, saponins and catechins, which can neutralize free radicals in the body.
- Red & white grape extracts - contain beneficial plant compounds, resveratrol, quercetin, anthocyanins and catechins - all combat the oxidative stress that can lead to illness.
- Grapefruit extract - contains many powerful antioxidants that can protect your body from oxidative stress and free radicals.
- Black carrot extract - is rich in anthocyanins which are powerful antioxidants.
- Vitamin B3 - is also known as Niacin. It helps the body convert food into glucose used for energy. Niacin supports the healthy function of the nervous system and normal psychological processes. It may also help ward off undue tiredness.

Slique® essential oil blend -
- Grapefruit rind oil - is naturally high in antioxidants and phytochemicals that reduce oxidative stress and inflammation. Limonene protects cells from damage.
- Tangerine rind oil - promotes good digestion while supporting the immune system.
- Spearmint leaf oil - promotes healthy digestion and acid secretion. Can also support the breakdown of food.
- Lemon rind oil - cleanses toxins from the body and stimulates lymphatic drainage.
- Ocotea leaf oil - has the highest levels of alpha-humulene in the world, known for its ability to minimize inflammation and irritation.
- Stevia leaf extract - is used as a natural sweetener, that has no accumulation in the body, which can promote healthy insulin production.

Vitamins and Minerals -
- Dipotassium phosphate - is commonly used as an emulsifier and is a great source of potassium and phosphorus.
- Monosodium phosphate - is used as an emulsifying agent and protein modifier. It is a good source of phosphorus, which is necessary for healthy bones.
- Magnesium oxide - is beneficial for the proper functioning of the immune system, nerves, heart, eyes, brain and muscles.
- Zinc gluconate - is important for growth and healthy development of body tissues.

Organic B vitamin blend -
- Guava extract - is rich in antioxidants, vitamin C, potassium and fiber and is used to make collagen, a protein required to help wounds heal.
- Holy basil extract - is an adaptogen with anti-inflammatory and antioxidant properties.
- Citrus limon extract - helps in the absorption of iron.

Other Ingredients -
- Alfalfa grass juice powder - has a high concentration of antioxidants, vitamins C and K, copper, folate and magnesium. It is also very low in calories.
- Organic wolfberry fruit powder - supports healthy vision thanks to high levels of an antioxidant called zeaxanthin. High amounts of Vitamins A and C build immunity and fight oxidative stressors.
- Stevia - a natural sweetener that is low in calories, derived from the Stevia leaf.
- Ascorbic acid - acts as an antioxidant, protecting cells from free radicals.
- Molybdenum glycinate - acts as a cofactor for the enzymes involved in processing sulfites and breaking down toxins in the body.
- Niacin (B3) - helps the body convert food into glucose, used for energy. Niacin supports the healthy function of the nervous system and normal psychological processes. It may also help ward off undue tiredness.
- Copper gluconate - helps the body form collagen, absorb iron and supports energy production.
- Biotin - is a water-soluble B vitamin that helps your body convert food into energy.
- Vitamin A acetate - is a powerful antioxidant necessary for eye health, immune function, cell growth and fetal development.
- Sodium selenite - is an essential trace mineral that plays an important role in reducing oxidative stress on the body.
- d-Calcium pantothenate - protects cells against damage by increasing levels of glutathione in the body.
- Chromium nicotinate glycinate chelate - is a high-quality, chelated form of the mineral chromium, an amino acid that binds to minerals and assists in their bioavailability through the intestinal walls.
- Riboflavin - is also known as Vitamin B2. It helps the break down of proteins, fats and carbohydrates. Riboflavin maintains the body's energy supply and converts carbohydrates into adenosine triphosphate (ATP), while absorbing and activating iron, folic acid, and vitamins B1, B3 and B6.
- Pyridoxine HCl - or vitamin B6, helps the body convert food into fuel, metabolize fats and proteins, maintain proper nerve functions and produce red blood cells.
- Potassium iodide - is stored in the thyroid gland and is necessary for normal function.
- Methylcobalamin - or B12, acts as a cofactor for enzymes, providing functional support of neurons. B12 can also reduce the neurotoxicity of cells.

COMMENTS FROM YOUNG LIVING

"Slique® Shake is a complete meal replacement that provides quick, satisfying, and delicious nutrition. Formulated with Slique® Essence essential oil blend, this shake may support healthy weight management when combined with regular exercise and a sensible diet. In a convenient single-serving size packet, it's easy to slip into a purse or pocket for healthy eating on the go."

DIRECTIONS FOR USE

Add 1 Slique® Shake packet to 8 ounces of water or the milk of your choice. Shake, stir, or blend until smooth.

SLIQUE® BARS *(Regular and Chocolate Coated)*

Simply put, Slique® Bars are delicious. Both the regular and chocolate coated are incredible! If you love the ease and taste of nut and fruit bars, you will instantly love these. They are the perfect mix of chewy, crunchy, and sweet. Eat a Slique® bar for breakfast or take with you as a midday snack. You will want to hide these from your kids! Mommy's special treat only!

INGREDIENTS

- Baru nuts
- Almonds
- Honey
- Chicory root inulin
- Dates,
- Coconut
- Cocao nib
- Goldenberries
- Bing cherries
- Wolfberries (Lycium barbarum)
- Quinoa crisps
- Chia seeds
- Potato skin extract
- Sea salt
- Vanilla (Vanilla planifolia) oil
- Sunflower lecithin
- Orange (Citrus aurantium dulcis) peel oil
- Cinnamon (Cinnamomum verum) bark oil.

Allergens - Contains baru nuts, almonds, and Coconut.
Manufactured in a facility that also processes tree nuts, peanuts, soy, milk, and eggs.

WHAT THE INGREDIENTS DO

- Baru nuts - high in fiber, protein, essential fatty acids and antioxidants.
- Almonds - high in protein, fiber, vitamin E, copper and magnesium.
- Honey - good source of antioxidants; beneficial to the cardiovascular system.
- Chicory root inulin - good source of prebiotic fiber; supports digestion and blood sugar.
- Dates - high in polyphenols, fiber, protein, B6, iron, and potassium.
- Coconut - may boost fat-burning and provide quick energy.
- Cocao nib - high in antioxidants, fiber, magnesium and iron; supports mood.
- Goldenberries - high in antioxidants, beta carotene and vitamin K; supports immunity.
- Bing cherries - high in antioxidants; supports cardiovascular and blood pressure levels.
- Wolfberries - high in antioxidants, vitamins and minerals; beneficial for eye, brain, skin and heart health; may assist with healthy blood sugar and cholesterol levels.
- Quinoa crisps - high in amino acids, fiber, B, calcium, iron, magnesium and phosphorus.
- Chia seeds - high in antioxidants, fiber, protein, iron, calcium and omega-3 fatty acids.
- Potato skin extract - natural antioxidant; increases the duration of satiety.
- Sea salt - good source of trace minerals; supports cardiovascular and electrolyte balance.
- Vanilla oil - high in antioxidants; curbs cravings.
- Sunflower lecithin - an emulsifier that supports brain, skin and digestive health.
- Orange peel oil - supports circulation, immunity, skin, and mood health; curbs cravings.
- Cinnamon Bark oil - high in antioxidants; supports immunity, circulation, and metabolism.

COMMENTS FROM YOUNG LIVING

"Members have always enjoyed Slique® Bars as a safe, delicious weight-management tool that utilizes a dual-target approach to help manage satiety. Now this innovative bar is coated in delicious dark chocolate! To support any weight-management plan, Slique® Bars are loaded with exotic baru nuts and wholesome almonds, which promote satiety when combined with protein and fiber. We also use a potato skin extract that, when ingested, triggers the release of cholecystokinin in the body, increasing the duration of feelings of fullness."

DIRECTIONS FOR USE

Consume before or between meals with 12 ounces of water to help control hunger.

The statements about the supplement and the ingredients have not been evaluated by the Food and Drug Administration. Young Living® products are not intended to diagnose, treat, cure, or prevent any disease.

SLIQUE® CITRASLIM™

Slique® CitraSlim™ is a great way to help support your metabolism and healthy weight. The ingredients help break down excess fat and help support a healthy appetite. This is recommended when using the full Slique® protocol or it may be used by itself for healthy weight maintenance.

INGREDIENTS
1 Liquid Capsule Ingredients - Proprietary Liquid Blend - 460 mg
- Lemongrass (Cymbopogon flexuosus) leaf oil
- Caprylic/capric glycerides
- Pomegranate (Punica granatum) seed oil
- Lemon myrtle (Backhousia citriodora) leaf oil
- Idaho Balsam fir (Abies balsamea) branch/leaf oil

Other Ingredients - Silicon dioxide, Gelatin, Water
Contains nut (coconut)

3 Powder Capsule Ingredients - Proprietary Powder Blend - 2088 mg
- Cassia (Cinnamomum cassia) dried bark powder
- Citrus based fruit blend - [Orange (Citrus sinesis) whole fruit extract, Grapefruit (Citrus Paradisi) whole fruit extract, Guarana (Paulinia cupana) whole fruit extract]
- Pterostilbene
- Bitter orange (Citrus aurantium) unripened fruit extract
- Ocotea (Ocotea quixos) leaf powder
- Fenugreek (Trigonella foenum-graecum) seed extract
- Digestive Enzymes - Amylase, Cellulase, Lipase, Protease
- Spearmint (Mentha spicata) leaf oil
- Ocotea (Ocotea quixos) leaf oil
- Cassia (Cinnamomum aromaticum) leaf oil
- Fennel (Foeniculum vulgare) seed oil

Other ingredients - Hypromellose, Rice Flour, Silicon dioxide.

WHAT THE INGREDIENTS DO
Liquid Capsule Ingredients -
- Lemongrass leaf oil - supports immunity and digestion.
- Caprylic/capric glycerides - from Coconut oil as a carrier base.
- Pomegranate seed oil - supports immunity, blood pressure, inflammation, and circulation.
- Lemon myrtle leaf oil - supports immunity and digestion.
- Idaho Balsam fir branch/leaf oil - soothes muscles and supports respiratory function.

3 Powder Capsule Ingredients -
- Cassia dried bark powder - helps support metabolism and immunity.
- Orange whole fruit extract - helps metabolize fat cells, supports immunity and circulation.
- Grapefruit whole fruit extract - helps metabolize fat cells.
- Guarana whole fruit extract - helps boost energy.
- Pterostilbene - supports healthy weight.
- Bitter orange unripened fruit extract - helps metabolize fat cells.
- Ocotea leaf powder - helps reduce blood sugars and supports sugar cravings.
- Fenugreek seed extract - supports digestion and improves exercise performance.

3 Powder Capsule Ingredients (continued)

Digestive Enzymes -
- Amylase - breaks down starch.
- Cellulase - breaks down cellulose (plant fiber).
- Lipase - breaks down dietary fats and oils, helps liver function.
- Protease - digests proteins and helps carries away toxins.

Essential Oils -
- Spearmint leaf oil - soothes digestion and promotes energy.
- Ocotea leaf oil - stimulates and optimizes digestion, helps lower blood sugar level, benefits cardiovascular health and promotes blood flow in the arteries and blood vessels, helps curb cravings and promote feelings of fullness, and stimulates the body to remove toxins through the liver.
- Cassia leaf oil - assists with nervous, digestive, circulatory and immune system health, and may assist with blood sugar balance.
- Fennel seed oil - supports digestion, metabolism, and fights free radical damage; helps relieve gas, bloating, and constipation; boosts metabolism while suppressing appetite.

Other ingredients - Hypromellose, Rice Flour, Silicon dioxide - capsule base and substrate.

COMMENTS FROM YOUNG LIVING

"Slique® CitraSlim™ is formulated with naturally derived ingredients to promote healthy weight management when combined with a balanced diet and regular exercise. Slique® CitraSlim™ also includes a proprietary citrus extract blend, which some studies suggest may help support the body in burning excess fat when used in conjunction with a healthy weight-management plan. This polyphenolic mixture of flavonoids offers powerful antioxidants that are touted for their health benefits. This blend may also support the release of free fatty acids, which help break down fat."

Once-Daily Liquid Capsule - The liquid capsule delivers pomegranate seed oil, Lemongrass, Lemon Myrtle, and Idaho Balsam Fir Essential Oils. This blend is high in citral, which is a constituent that may increase metabolic activity.

Powder Capsules - Three power-packed powder capsules contain a proprietary citrus extract blend, cinnamon powder, bitter orange extract, fenugreek seed, ocotea leaf extract, and a customized blend of enzymes and four Essential Oils - Ocotea, Cassia, Spearmint, and Fennel.

DIRECTIONS FOR USE

Consume 2 powder capsules in the morning with 8 ounces of water. Consume 1 powder and 1 liquid capsule with 8 ounces of water in the afternoon, before 3 p.m. If you miss taking your capsules in the morning, you may take all 4 capsules together in the afternoon, before 3 p.m.

The statements about the supplement and the ingredients have not been evaluated by the Food and Drug Administration. Young Living® products are not intended to diagnose, treat, cure, or prevent any disease.

SLIQUE® GUM

Slique® Gum is not your traditional gum. Take a step back to ancient times when people would chew on gum resins to help clean their teeth and gums and also curb their appetite. The gum tablet starts off as a slight powder and transforms in your mouth to a short-term chewing gum to help keep your cravings at bay. Chew one tablet in the afternoon when your cravings are at their highest. Drink lots of water or have a glass of Slique® Tea to support afternoon cravings as well.

INGREDIENTS
- Frankincense Resin (Boswellia frereana)
- Gumbase
- Isomalt
- Sorbitol
- Natural Flavors
- Calcium Stearate
- Natural Sweeteners
- Red Cabbage Juice
- Turmeric

Slimming Fresh Mint Essential Oil Blend -
- Peppermint (Mentha Piperita) Oil
- Spearmint (Mentha Spicata) Leaf Oil
- Xylitol

Allergens - Contains Traces of Soy. No artificial Colors of Flavors.

WHAT THE INGREDIENTS DO
- Frankincense Resin - strengthens teeth and gums and is beneficial to oral health.
- Gumbase - proprietary industry formula made from several food-grade raw materials.
- Isomalt - naturally sourced sugar-free sugar replacement made from beet sugar.
- Sorbitol - low calorie fruit-derived sugar.
- Calcium Stearate - calcium combined with vegetable oil used to thicken and stabilize.
- Natural Sweeteners - to enhance experience and natural colors from
- Red Cabbage Juice - for color.
- Turmeric - for color.

Slimming Fresh Mint Essential Oil Blend -
- Peppermint Oil - supports digestive health, stimulates brain function, immune boosting benefits, promotes energy and focus and uplifts emotions.
- Spearmint Leaf Oil - soothes digestion, promotes energy and is emotionally uplifting.
- Xylitol - naturally occurring plant-based sugar alcohol (not for dogs).

COMMENTS FROM YOUNG LIVING
"Ancient travelers throughout the Middle East used raw frankincense resin for its nutritional content and ability to help control hunger. Slique® Gum offers those same benefits in a modern delivery system that helps control food cravings and improve oral health."

DIRECTIONS FOR USE
Chewing 1 gum tablet before or after meals or as desired may help control cravings. CAUTION: Keep away from dogs due to xylitol.

The statements about the supplement and the ingredients have not been evaluated by the Food and Drug Administration. Young Living® products are not intended to diagnose, treat, cure, or prevent any disease.

SLIQUE® ESSENCE ESSENTIAL OIL

Slique® Essence essential oil blend is the perfect addition to your healthy weight loss goals. A few drops per day is all that is needed. Simply add 1-2 drops to a glass or stainless steel water bottle and fill with cold water. Sip throughout the day to get the cleansing benefits of this blend. Slique® Essence adds a refreshing citrus flavor to your water, which helps you drink more water without all the added sugar and chemicals found in store brand flavored waters.

INGREDIENTS
- Grapefruit (Citrus paradisi) rind oil
- Tangerine (Citrus reticulata) rind oil
- Spearmint (Mentha spicata) leaf oil
- Lemon (Citrus limon) rind oil
- Ocotea (Ocotea quixos) leaf oil
- Stevia (Rebaudiana) leaf extract

WHAT THE INGREDIENTS DO
- Grapefruit rind oil - boosts metabolism, stimulates the lymphatic system, supports detoxification and digestion, helps reduce sugar cravings, balances blood sugar levels, and reduces your appetite.
- Tangerine rind oil - relaxes nerves and muscles, and reduces tension, helps the body remove toxins, supports the digestive system and speeds up the metabolism.
- Spearmint leaf oil - relieves gas and indigestion and improves digestion.
- Lemon rind oil - improves digestion, supports metabolism, and cleanses the lymphatic glands. Stimulates lymphatic drainage for toxin removal. Promotes detoxification through the blood and liver. Reduces oxidative stress. Helps boost the immune system.
- Ocotea leaf oil - stimulates and optimizes digestion, helps lower blood sugar levels, supports cardiovascular health, and promotes blood flow in the arteries and blood vessels. Helps curb cravings and promote feelings of fullness. Helps curb sugar cravings.
- Stevia leaf extract - provides sweetness with zero calories.

COMMENTS FROM YOUNG LIVING
"Slique® Essence combines Grapefruit, Tangerine, Lemon, Spearmint, and Ocotea with stevia extract in a unique blend that supports healthy weight management goals. These ingredients work together to help control hunger, especially when used in conjunction with Slique® Tea or the Slique® Kit. The pleasant citrus combination of Grapefruit, Tangerine, and Lemon essential oils adds a flavorful and uplifting element to any day with the added support of Spearmint that may help with digestion. Ocotea essential oil adds an irresistible, cinnamon-like aroma to help control hunger, while stevia adds an all-natural sweetener that provides a pleasant taste with no added calories."

DIRECTIONS FOR USE
Shake vigorously before use. Add 2-4 drops to 4-6 oz. of your favorite beverage, Slique® Tea, or water. Use between and during meals regularly throughout the day whenever hunger feelings occur.

Aromatic - Direct inhalation preferred.
Note - Stevia extract in this formula may impede diffuser performance.

The statements about the supplement and the ingredients have not been evaluated by the Food and Drug Administration. Young Living® products are not intended to diagnose, treat, cure, or prevent any disease.

SULFURZYME® *(Capsules & Powder)*

Healthier hair, smoother skin, stronger nails? Yes please! How about cells that regenerate themselves cleaner and stronger for better mobility? And how about a more stable immune system and circulatory system? Yes, yes, and yes! Oh and can I please have a better supported liver to cleanse and filter my blood and help detox my system? Also I'd like something that will help detox my whole body and give me more energy. Why of course! You get all of these benefits plus more with adding organic natural sulfur amino acids to your diet.

Sulfur is responsible for vital amino acids in our body that support healthy cells, skin, hormones, and enzymes. Sulfur is naturally found in all plant and animal cells. Sulfur amino acids help our body produce glutathione. Glutathione increases energy, improves mental clarity and focus, helps support proper immune function, improves the quality of sleep, supports athletic recovery, slows down the aging process, detoxifies the cells and liver, increases keratin production in skin, hair, and nails, plus more!

Many people claim they have a sulfur allergy. This is incorrect. People cannot be allergic to sulfur as that would be like saying you are allergic to water. Sulfa is commonly mixed up with sulfur and also doctors may refer to "sulfur allergies", but they mean specifically the pharmaceutical called sulfonamide. In an article by William B. Smith and Constance H. Katelaris of the Australian Prescriber entitled "'Sulfur allergy' label is misleading" they state, "Many patients believe that having been labelled 'sulfur allergic' they are also at risk of adverse reactions or allergies from sulfites, sulfates and even elemental sulfur and may attempt to avoid them. ... Patients who have had allergic reactions to sulfonamide drugs do not need to avoid sulfites, sulfates or sulfur."

Sulfurzyme® powder contains a natural organic form of dietary sulfur. The wolfberries in Sulfurzyme® have a dual action to help allow the MSM to be more bioavailable by allowing it to be more readily assimilated and metabolized by the body. Wolfberries are also an excellent source of prebiotics. Both the powder and the capsules contain prebiotics, but the powder contains even more in the form of Fructooligosaccharides.

RECIPES

The NingXia Daily Boost - Try adding 1/2 teaspoon (I use a full teaspoon so adjust accordingly) of Sulfurzyme® power to 2 ounces of NingXia Red® and one tube of NingXia NITRO® in the morning for 30 days instead of your morning coffee and you'll feel a big difference.

The Red Drink by Dr. Peter Minke - 2 ounces NingXia Red®, ½ teaspoon Sulfurzyme®, 16-32 ounces of water, and 3 drops of Lime Vitality™.

Note on allergies. If you are allergic to sulfa, you won't be allergic to sulfur. Your body naturally produces sulfur, so rest assured, using a supplemental form of organic dietary MSM (Methylsulfonylmethane) such as Sulfurzyme®, is a great way to support your overall health.

SULFURZYME® *(Capsules)*

INGREDIENTS
Proprietary Sulfurzyme® Blend - 1.8 g
- Wolfberry fruit powder (prebiotic)
- MSM - Methylsulfonylmethane (an organic form of dietary sulfur)

WHAT THE INGREDIENTS DO
- MSM - protects cells and replenishes the connection between cells. Supports joint pain, inflammation, increases glutathione levels, helps speed up post-exercise recovery, supports the reduction of pain and joint stiffness, improves flexibility, strengthens hair and nails, improves complexion and skin, provides natural energy increase, helps detox the body.
- Wolfberry fruit powder - prebiotic that supports gut health; supports the bioavailability of MSM; a natural polysaccharide that supports the healthy function of the immune system, as well as healthy regeneration of tissues and cells.

Other Ingredients - Hypromellose, Rice Flour, Magnesium stearate, Silica (capsule and substrate).

SULFURZYME® *(Powder)*

INGREDIENTS
Calcium 8 g
Proprietary Sulfurzyme® Powder Blend - 2.02 g
- Wolfberry fruit powder (prebiotic)
- MSM - Methylsulfonylmethane (an organic form of dietary sulfur)
- FOS Fructooligosaccharides prebiotic

Other Ingredients - Stevia (Stevia rebaudiana) leaf extract, and Calcium Silicate

WHAT THE INGREDIENTS DO
- Calcium - supports healthy bones and provides supplement base.
- MSM - protects cells and replenishes the connection between cells. Supports joint pain, inflammation, increases glutathione levels, helps speed up post-exercise recovery, supports the reduction of pain and joint stiffness, improves flexibility, strengthens hair and nails, improves complexion and skin, provides natural energy increase, helps detox the body.
- Wolfberry fruit powder - prebiotic that supports gut health; supports the bioavailability of MSM; a natural polysaccharide that supports the healthy function of the immune system, as well as healthy regeneration of tissues and cells.
- FOS - prebiotic that feeds the good flora in your gut.

Other Ingredients - Stevia leaf extract - natural sweetener. Calcium Silicate - anti-caking agent.

COMMENTS FROM YOUNG LIVING
Sulfurzyme® combines wolfberry with MSM, a naturally occurring organic form of dietary sulfur needed by our bodies every day to maintain the structure of proteins, protect cells and cell membranes, replenish the connections between cells, and preserve the molecular framework of connective tissue. MSM also supports the immune system, the liver, circulation, and proper intestinal function and works to scavenge free radicals. Wolfberries contain minerals and coenzymes that support the assimilation and metabolism of sulfur. FOS is added to this formula to support normal digestive system health."

DIRECTIONS FOR USE
Capsules: Take 2 capsules twice daily in between meals for optimal results.
Powder: Mix 1/2 teaspoon with juice or distilled water and take twice daily, one hour before or after meals.

SUPER B™

Young Living's Super B™ contains all eight B vitamins - B1, B2, B3, B5, B6, B7, B9, and B12. That is why it is called SUPER B™! B vitamins help keep our cells metabolizing correctly. They are water soluble and are helpful to support normal energy levels. They have a whole host of benefits. Read below on each B Vitamin and their benefits. Super B™ is infused with Nutmeg essential oil which is known for its energy enhancing qualities.

INGREDIENTS
- B1 Thiamin (as thiamin HCI) 1670% (25 mg)
- B2 Riboflavin 1470% (25 mg)
- B3 Niacin (nicotinic acid and niacinamide) 180% (35 mg)
- B5 Pantothenic acid (as d-calcium pantothenate) 150% (15 mg)
- B6 (pyridoxine HCI) 1250% (25 mg)
- B7 Biotin (Vitamin H) 50% (150 mcg)
- B9 Folate 100% (400 mcg)
- B12 (methylcobalamin) 1670% (100 mcg)
- Calcium (as dicalcium phosphate) 143 mg
- Magnesium (as magnesium bisglycinate chelate) 10 mg
- Zinc (as zinc bisglycinate chelate) 3 mg
- Selenium (as selenium glycinate complex) 50 mcg
- Manganese (as manganese bisglycinate chelate) 0.5 mg

Proprietary Super B™ Blend - 30 mg
- PABA (Para amino benzoic acid), Nutmeg (Myristica fragrans) seed oil

WHAT THE INGREDIENTS DO
- B1 (Thiamine) - supports a healthy nervous system and helps improve cardiovascular function. It helps to break down fats and proteins. B1 helps convert carbohydrates into glucose to help give energy to the body to perform various functions. It also helps the body withstand stress and maintain a healthy metabolism.
- B2 (Riboflavin) - helps the body break down proteins, fats, and carbohydrates to produce energy. It is a powerful anti-inflammatory that is known to support brain, bone, and eye health. It also supports the liver, blood pressure, and the cardiovascular system. B2 may also support positive moods. It ma of nighttime leg cramps in the elderly as well as healthier pregnancies.
- B3 (Niacin) - is known to help lower cholesterol, increase brain function, support mood swings, help with skin issues, support mental clarity and memory, as well as ease arthritis symptoms. It is important not to take too much Niacin as you can experience what is known as a Niacin flush. Overdosing (250 milligrams or more) on Niacin is uncomfortable but will not harm you. The amount in Super B™ is a good adult amount for daily supplementation.
- B5 (Pantothenic acid) - helps support a healthy metabolism and other bodily functions. It helps convert the food you eat into energy. It works as an anti-inflammatory and supports the immune, nervous, and gastrointestinal systems. B5 is also known to help balance cholesterol levels and reduce stress.
- B6 (Pyridoxine) - is a helpful supplement to support healthy emotions. It works in the brain to provide healthier cognition. It has been studied to reduce heart disease risk, help aid in hemoglobin production, and support PMS symptoms. It is also used to help nausea during pregnancy. B6 supports the digestive tract, heart health, and muscle function.
- B7 (Biotin or Vitamin H) - helps convert fat, protein, and carbohydrates into energy. This vitamin is important to use if you are pregnant or breast-feeding. It has been touted as a supplement to support healthy hair, skin, and nails.

- B9 (Folate) - not folic acid. Folic acid is often labeled as B9 but it is the lesser synthetic version of folate. You should always look for folate over folic acid. Folate is needed for your body to make DNA. Having enough folate may prevent iron deficiency. It helps promote hair, skin and nail health through cell regeneration. Folate is an important supplement for pregnant women to help prevent certain birth defects. It is also noted that folate supports your mood by transforming amino acids from your food into neurotransmitters such as serotonin and dopamine.
- B12 (Methylcobalamin) - plays an important role in helping you make red blood cells. It is known as the "painkilling vitamin". It supports brain health, eye health, skin health, DNA production, cardiovascular support, and converts the food you eat into energy. It also supports improved sleep-wake patterns as well as healthy emotions. There are several forms of B12 and Methylcobalamin is the most bioavailable of all forms of B12.
- Calcium (dicalcium phosphate) - helps prevent bone loss and repairs joints.
- Magnesium - aids in normal function of the cells, nerves, muscles, bones, and heart.
- Zinc (as zinc bisglycinate chelate) - highly absorbable form of zinc.
- Selenium - is a powerful antioxidant that defends against free radicals in the body.
- Manganese - supports metabolism, blood sugar, and PMS cramps.

Proprietary Super B™ Blend - 30 mg
- PABA (Para amino benzoic acid) - supports skin elasticity, hair loss and color, and joints.
- Nutmeg seed oil - supports lymphatic, digestive, and immune health; promotes energy.

COMMENTS FROM YOUNG LIVING

"Super B™ is a comprehensive vitamin complex containing all eight essential, energy-boosting B vitamins (B1, B2, B3, B5, B6, B7, B9, and B12). Recently reformulated, it now features Orgen-FA®, a natural folate source derived from lemon peels, and methylcobalamin, a more bioavailable source of B12. Combined with Nutmeg essential oil and bioavailable chelated minerals such as magnesium, manganese, selenium, and zinc, Super B™ not only assists in maintaining healthy energy levels, but it also supports mood and cardiovascular and cognitive function. B vitamins are essential to our health and well-being, and each B vitamin performs a unique and separate function in the body. Unfortunately, they must be replenished daily, as they are not stored in the body."

DIRECTIONS FOR USE

Two tablets first thing in the morning 30 minutes before breakfast. It is best to split the dose by taking one tablet in the morning 30 minutes before breakfast and one tablet 30 minutes before lunch. This may also be taken with breakfast and lunch, but is water soluble so it is not necessary to take with food. Do not take in the evening as this may cause insomnia or restlessness. If it upsets your stomach you may take it with a little food or try taking half a tablet.

Note: this supplement will turn your urine bright yellow. This is normal.

The statements about the supplement and the ingredients have not been evaluated by the Food and Drug Administration. Young Living® products are not intended to diagnose, treat, cure, or prevent any disease.

SUPER C™ *(Chewables & Tablets)*

Vitamin C is something we need daily, as our bodies do not produce it on its own. The benefits of vitamin C are varied, but most of us consider it a wonderful way to strengthen our immune system. Vitamin C has also been touted as a way to support the cardiovascular system, help with prenatal care, support healthy eye function, and skin smoothing! Yes, our favorite vitamin C can help you look younger. When you use isolated Vitamin C you are only getting a small amount of its intended benefits. Vitamin C works best when it is consumed as the whole fruit. Fruit purchased at the grocery store is depleted of vital nutrients as they were often picked two weeks prior to you receiving them. Vine-ripening is the best form of whole-fruit nutrition, but if you do not live on or near a farm that allows you to pick ripe fruit and eat it the same day, then you are eating vitamin depleted fruit.

Bioflavonoids are a key part of the whole fruit. They help enhance vitamin C action and are known to support blood circulation and help decrease free-radical damage in the body. Because they are so good at placating anti-oxidative stress, they are able to help support inflammatory conditions in the body. Super C™ from Young Living® allows you to get all the benefits of vine-ripened fruit with all the beautiful bioflavonoids without traveling to a farm or becoming an orchard owner of five varieties of citrus. While some of you have access to these, the majority of us do not. There are two Super C™ products from which to choose in the Young Living® supplement line; tablets and chewable. They are a bit different, so take a look at both to determine your needs.

SUPER C™ *(Chewables)*

Super C™ Chewables contain whole fruit powder from five different citrus fruits. These contain powerful bioflavonoids and are sourced from Lemon, Orange, Lime, Tangerine, and Grapefruit. Using the whole fruit that is juiced and then dried to form a powder ensures you get the full botanical synergy of the vitamins. The Chewable also contains Acerola fruit extract, Camu camu whole fruit powder, Rose hips fruit powder and Orange peel oil powder. This vitamin C supplement is a powerful way to support your health!

INGREDIENTS
Calories 5
Carbohydrates (Sugars) 1g
- Vitamin C (as ascorbic acid) 150 mg (170% DV)

Proprietary Super C™ Blend - 460 mg
- Acerola (Malpighia glabra) fruit extract
- Camu camu (Myrciaria dubia) whole fruit powder
- Rose hips (Rosa canina) fruit powder

Citrus bioflavonoids -
- Lemon (Citrus limon) whole fruit powder
- Orange (Citrus sinensis) whole fruit powder
- Lime (Citrus Aurantifolia) whole fruit powder
- Tangerine (Citrus reticulata) whole fruit powder
- Grapefruit (Citrus paradisi) whole fruit powder.
- Orange (Citrus sinesis) peel oil powder.

Other Ingredients - Non-GMO Tapioca dextrose, Sorbitol, Calcium ascorbate, Stevia, Hydroxypropyl cellulose, Stearic acid, Silicon dioxide, Magnesium stearate.

WHAT THE INGREDIENTS DO

- Ascorbic Acid (Vitamin C) - acts as an antioxidant, protecting cells from free radicals.
- Acerola fruit extract - an antioxidant nutrient, rich in vitamin C.
- Camu camu whole fruit powder - contains powerful antioxidants, including anthocyanins and ellagic acid, is high in vitamin C and may fight inflammation.
- Rose hips fruit powder - contains antioxidants that are anti-inflammatory, protect immune cells from oxidative stress and encourage white blood cell production.
- Orange peel oil powder - contains Limonene, which is a monocyclic, monoterpene that defends against oxidative stress that can negatively affect the immune system.

Citrus bioflavonoids - support the immune system and enhance the action of vitamin C, promote healthy blood circulation and work to reduce inflammation in the body.
- Orange whole fruit powder - a concentrated source of Vitamin C, which doubles as a powerful antioxidant and plays a central role in immune function.
- Lime whole fruit powder - boosts iron absorption, supports healthy blood sugar and cholesterol levels.
- Tangerine whole fruit powder - contains beneficial compounds with anti-inflammatory properties, aiding in the digestion of fatty foods.
- Grapefruit whole fruit powder - is rich in nutrients, antioxidants and fiber. It provides vitamins A and C, folate (B9), choline, limonins and lycopene.

Other Ingredients -
- Non-GMO Tapioca dextrose - simple, easily digested sugar.
- Sorbitol - low calorie fruit-derived sugar.
- Calcium ascorbate - easily digested form of C.
- Stevia - no-calorie sweetener.
- Hydroxypropyl cellulose - tablet binder.
- Stearic acid - ingredient binder.
- Silicon dioxide - natural anti-caking agent.
- Magnesium stearate - helps lubricate the tablets.

COMMENTS FROM YOUNG LIVING

"Super C™ combines pure Orange essential oil with a proprietary blend of camu camu, acerola, cherry, and rose hips fruit powder to create a powerful immune-supporting supplement. Together, these premium ingredients deliver desirable polyphenols, carotenoids, and optimal amounts of vitamin C in a convenient chewable tablet."

DIRECTIONS FOR USE

Take daily or when additional vitamin C is desired.
Take 1 chewable tablet 3 times daily or as needed.

The statements about the supplement and the ingredients have not been evaluated by the Food and Drug Administration. Young Living® products are not intended to diagnose, treat, cure, or prevent any disease.

SUPER C™ *(Tablets)*

Super C™ Tablets differ from the Chewables in that they contain Rutin flower bud powder, Cayenne fruit powder, Orange peel oil, Tangerine rind oil, Grapefruit peel oil, Lemon peel oil, and Lemongrass leaf oil. The tablets do not contain the whole-fruit powders of Orange, Lime, Tangerine, Grapefruit, and Camu camu that are found in the chewables. Instead, it contains the essential oils that allow for better bioavailability of the ingredients and the added benefits of dicalcium phosphate, zinc, manganese, and potassium.

INGREDIENTS
Calories 5
Carbohydrates 2 g
- Vitamin C (as ascorbic acid) 1.3 g (1440% DV)
- Calcium (calcium carbonate and dicalcium phosphate) 160 mg (10% DV)
- Zinc (as zinc gluconate) 1 mg (10% DV)
- Manganese (as manganese sulfate) 2 mg (90% DV)
- Potassium (as potassium chloride) 20 mg (<1% DV)

Proprietary Super C™ Blend - 78 mg
- Citrus bioflavonoids
- Rutin (Sophora japonica L) flower bud powder
- Cayenne (Capsicum annuum) fruit powder
- Orange (Citrus sinensis) peel oil
- Tangerine (Citrus reticulata) rind oil
- Grapefruit (Citrus paradisi) peel oil
- Lemon (Citrus limon) peel oil
- Lemongrass (Cymbopogon flexuosus) leaf oil

WHAT THE INGREDIENTS DO
- Ascorbic Acid (Vitamin C) - acts as an antioxidant, protecting cells from free radicals.
- Calcium - supports bone health, muscle contractions, and weight maintenance.
- Zinc - promotes a healthy immune system. Aids in healing of wounds.
- Manganese (as manganese sulfate) - supports nutrient absorption and bone health.
- Potassium (as potassium chloride) - used to maintain fluid and electrolyte balance.
- Citrus Bioflavonoids - help maximize the benefits of vitamin C.
- Rutin flower bud powder - antioxidant; supports circulation and blood vessels.
- Cayenne fruit powder - supports digestion, cramps, circulation, metabolism, and digestion.
- Orange peel oil - supports immune system, improves blood flow, and anti-inflammatory.
- Tangerine rind oil - reduces acne, brightens skin, reduces oily skin, and diminishes wrinkles.
- Grapefruit peel oil - supports fat burning and sugar cravings.
- Lemon peel oil - cleanses toxins from body, stimulates lymphatic drain, and purifies the skin.
- Lemongrass leaf oil - supports immune and lymphatic systems.

COMMENTS FROM YOUNG LIVING
"Super C™ not only contains 1440% of the recommended dietary intake of vitamin C per serving, but it is also fortified with rutin, citrus bioflavonoids, and minerals to balance electrolytes and enhance the effectiveness and absorption of vitamin C. The essential oils that are added may also increase bioflavonoid activity."

DIRECTIONS FOR USE
For reinforcing immune strength, take 2 tablets daily.
For maintenance, take 1 tablet daily. Best if taken before meals.

The statements about the supplement and the ingredients have not been evaluated by the Food and Drug Administration. Young Living® products are not intended to diagnose, treat, cure, or prevent any disease.

SUPER CAL™ PLUS

Start your morning off with supporting those bones! Eat a little something with these because it needs a little fat to get into your system. Even just a handful of nuts is good. This is not your mother's calcium supplement. Oh no! They are far better and so much more bioavailable. You will absolutely love these. They should become a part of your daily regimen for sure.

INGREDIENTS

- Vitamin D (D3 as cholecalciferol) 10 mcg
- Vitamin K (K2 as menquinone-7) 33 mg
- Calcium 260 mg
- Magnesium (as magnesium citrate) 119 mg

Super Cal™ Plus Dual Action Blend 1134 mg
- Marine minerals, Fermented polysaccharide complex, L-Lysine, L-Arginine, Winged treebine (Cissus quadrangularis) root extract PE 2.5%, Hops (Humulus lupulus) flower extract PE 4 -1, Tea (Camellia sinensis) leaf extract

Super Cal™ Plus Essential Oil Blend 5.5 mg
- Idaho Blue Spruce (Picea pungens) wood/branch/leaf oil, Black spruce (Picea mariana) wood/branches/needle oil, Copaiba (oleoresin) (Copaifera officinalis) wood oil, Vetiver (Vetiveria zizanoides) root oil, Peppermint (Mentha piperita) aerial parts oil.

Other Ingredients - Stearic acid, Non-GMO corn starch, Gelatin

WHAT THE INGREDIENTS DO

- Vitamin D - supports healthy bones and helps support immunity.
- Vitamin K - helps to push calcium into the bones.
- Calcium - helps prevent bone loss.
- Magnesium - supports the immune system, nerves, heart, eyes, brain, and muscles.

Super Cal™ Plus Dual Action Blend -
- Marine minerals: supports tissues and bones; helps maintain fluid and pH balance.

Fermented polysaccharide complex -
- L-lysine - converts fatty acids into energy; supports absorption of calcium; supports stress.
- L-arginine - stimulates the release of hormones and insulin, promotes increased blood flow.
- Winged treebine root extract - supports blood and heart health.
- Hops flower extract - helps to maintain a healthy weight by fighting oxidative stress.
- Tea leaf extract - supports blood, skin, liver, and brain health.

Super Cal™ Plus Essential Oil Blend -
- Idaho Blue Spruce oil - contains high amounts of alpha-pinene and limonene for bone health.
- Black spruce oil - alpha-pinene, camphene, and beta-pinene for bone and muscle health.
- Copaiba oil - supports inflammatory response in muscles and joints.
- Vetiver oil - supports joints and skin.
- Peppermint oil - supports bones, muscles, joints, and ligaments.

COMMENTS FROM YOUNG LIVING

"Using a marine mineral blend derived from red algae that's harvested off the coast of Iceland, Super Cal™ Plus harnesses the power of naturally derived ingredients to bring you the vital minerals found in the most complete bone-support supplement. This unique seaweed absorbs calcium, magnesium, and other trace minerals from ocean water, bringing them together to support overall bone health, including bone-density support."

DIRECTIONS FOR USE

Take 2 capsules daily with food.

The statements about the supplement and the ingredients have not been evaluated by the Food and Drug Administration. Young Living® products are not intended to diagnose, treat, cure, or prevent any disease.

THYROMIN™

Thyromin™ is a glandular supplement containing bovine (cow) thyroid powder, porcine (pig) pituitary powder, and porcine (pig) adrenal powder. These work well for those with poor functioning thyroids because the extracts contain active hormones. Thyromin™ is an excellent alternative for those who wish to support their thyroid and adrenals in a more natural way. Many medical doctors are now seeing the greater benefits to prescribing bovine and porcine glandular supplements over the traditional synthetic counterparts.

Many older research claims online have a negative view simply because there was not enough data. As more and more people are seeing major benefits from glandular supplementation, the newer articles are changing to reflect a more positive view. As you research this on your own, it is recommended that you check the date of the article and only look at more recent studies and reviews.

INGREDIENTS
- Vitamin E as mixed tocopherols (10 mg)
- Iodine from whole plant Kelp and potassium iodide (547 mcg)

Thyromin™ Blend
- Parsley leaf powder
- Bovine Thyroid powder (cow)
- Pituitary powder from porcine (pig)
- Adrenal powder from porcine (pig)
- L-Tyrosine
- L-Cystine
- L-Cysteine HCL
- Essential oils - Peppermint, Spearmint, Myrtle, Myrrh

WHAT THE INGREDIENTS DO
- Vitamin E - high antioxidant property.
- Iodine - needed to make thyroid hormone.
- Parsley leaf powder - improves digestion, and helps promote menstrual flow.
- Bovine Thyroid powder (cow) - helps to replace missing or lacking thyroid hormones.
- Pituitary powder from porcine (pig) - helps to replace missing or lacking pituitary hormones.
- Adrenal powder from porcine (pig) - helps to replace missing or lacking adrenal hormones.
- L-Tyrosine - an amino acid that helps improve mental performance, alertness, and memory.
- L-Cystine - an amino acid that is the basic building block of glutathione, for longevity, liver detoxification, and cognitive health. Helps fight oxidative stress.
- L-Cysteine HCL - supports anti-aging properties in cells; supports the immune system.
- Essential oils - Peppermint, Spearmint, Myrtle, Myrrh - makes ingredients more bioavailable.

COMMENTS FROM YOUNG LIVING
"Thyromin™ is a special blend of porcine glandular extracts, herbs, amino acids, minerals, and therapeutic-grade essential oils in a perfectly balanced formula that maximizes nutritional support for healthy thyroid function. The thyroid gland regulates body metabolism, energy, and body temperature."

DIRECTIONS FOR USE
Take 1-2 capsules daily, immediately before going to sleep.

The statements about the supplement and the ingredients have not been evaluated by the Food and Drug Administration. Young Living® products are not intended to diagnose, treat, cure, or prevent any disease.

SECTION THREE
the ingredients

NOTES:

VITAMINS

A (Beta-carotene) Fat Soluble
- Master Formula™ 100% DV (500 IU)
- Master Formula™ 90% DV (4500 IU)
- Balance Complete™ 25%
- KidScents® MightyVites™ 180 mcg

B1 (Thiamin) Water Soluble
- Master Formula™ 730% DV (11 mg)
- Super B™ 1670% DV (25 mg)
- Balance Complete™ 25%
- Pure Protein™ Complete 50% DV (0.75 mg)
- KidScents® MightyVites™ 0.8 mg

B2 (Riboflavin) Water Soluble
- Master Formula™ 590% DV (10 mg)
- Super B™ 1470% DV (25 mg)
- Balance Complete™ 25%
- Pure Protein™ Complete 50% DV (0.85 mg)
- KidScents® MightyVites™ 0.9 mg

B3 (Niacin) Water Soluble
- Master Formula™ 90% DV (17 mg)
- Super B™ 180% (35 mg)
- Balance Complete™ 30%
- Pure Protein™ Complete 50% DV (10 mg)
- KidScents® MightyVites™ 9 mg

B5 (Pantothenic acid) Water Soluble
- Master Formula™ 190% DV (19 mg)
- Mineral Essence™ ionic trace amounts
- Super B™ 150% DV (15 mg)
- Balance Complete™ 25%
- KidScents® MightyVites™ 1.8 mg

B6 (Pyridoxine) Water Soluble
- Master Formula™ 550% DV (11 mg)
- Mineral Essence™ ionic trace amounts
- Super B™ 1250% DV (25 mg)
- Balance Complete™ 25%
- Pure Protein™ Complete 50% DV (1 mg)
- EndoGize™ 1470% (25 mg)
- PowerGize™ 12 mg
- KidScents® MightyVites™ 2.2 mg

B7 (Biotin or Vitamin H) Water Soluble
- Master Formula™ 100% DV (300 mcg)
- Super B™ 50% DV (150 mg)
- Balance Complete™ 30%
- Pure Protein™ Complete 50% DV (150 mcg)
- KidScents® MightyVites™ 40 mcg

B9 (Folate. NOT Folic Acid) Water Soluble
- Master Formula™ 90% DV (350 mcg)
- Super B™ 100% DV (150 mcg)
- Balance Complete™ 30%
- KidScents® MightyVites™ 90 mcg DFE
- CardoGize 41% DV (165 mcg DFE)

B12 (Methylcobalamin) Water Soluble
- Master Formula™ 200% DV (12 mcg)
- Super B™ 1670% DV (100 mcg)
- Balance Complete™ 35%
- Pure Protein™ Complete 50% DV (3 mcg)
- KidScents® MightyVites™ 3.2 mcg

NOTES:

NOTES:

C Water Soluble
- MegaCal™ 15 % DV (9 mg)
- KidScents® MightyVites™ 27 mg
- Slique® Bar Tropical Berry 15%

C (Ascorbic Acid) Water Soluble
- Super C™ Chewable 170% DV (150 mg)
- Super C™ Tablets 1440% DV (1.3 g)
- Balance Complete™ 25%

C (Calcium Ascorbate) Water Soluble
- Master Formula™ 100% DV (61 mg)
- MegaCal™
- Super C™ Chewable

D3 (Cholecalciferol) Fat Soluble
- Master Formula™ 100% DV
- Super Cal™ Plus 10 mcg
- OmegaGize3™ 120 % DV (24 mcg)
- MindWise™ 100% DV (20 mcg)
- KidScents® MightyVites™ 5 mcg
- Balance Complete™ 25%

E Fat Soluble
- AminoWise™ 1.2 mg
- Master Formula™ 170% DV
- Balance Complete™ 15%
- Thyromin™ 67% DV (10 mg)
- KidScents® MightyVites™ 30 mg

Folic Acid
- Balance Complete™

K2 Fat Soluble
- Master Formula™ 60% DV
- Super Cal™ Plus 33 mg
- CardioGize™ 80% DV (100 mcg)

MINERALS

Beta-Carotene
- Balance Complete™ 25%

Black Pepper Fruit Extract
- EndoGize™ 448 mg

Boron
- Mineral Essence™ ionic trace amounts

Calcium
- Super Cal™ Plus 260 mg
- ICP™ 2% (14 mg)
- Slique® Bar Tropical Berry 2%
- NingXia Red® 4% (40 mg)

Calcium (Red Algae)
- Super Cal™ Plus 260 mg

Calcium Ascorbate
- MegaCal™ 20% DV (207 mg)
- Super C™ chewable

Calcium Carbonate
- Master Formula™ 20% DV (200 mg)
- ICP™ 14mg/serving
- Super C™ Tablets 10% DV (160 mg)
- Life 9™ 4% DV (63.9 mg)
- KidScents® MightyZyme™ 50mg
- Sulfurzyme® Powder 8 g
- AlkaLime 15% DV (201 mg)
- ImmuPro™ 6% (84 mg)
- MegalCal 20% DV (207 mg)

Calcium Citrate
- AminoWise™ 277 mg

Calcium (Dicalcium Phosphate)
- Super B™ 15% DV (143 mg)
- Super C™ Tablets 10% DV (160 mg)
- Pure Protein™ Complete 10% DV (100 mg)
- Essentialzyme™ 6% DV (70 mg)
- AlkaLime 15% DV (201 mg)
- JuvaTone® 35% DV (344 mg)

Calcium Fructoborate
- AgilEase™

NOTES:

NOTES:

Calcium Glycerophosphate
- MegaCal™ 20% DV (207 mg)

Calcium Lactate
- MegaCal™ 20% DV (207 mg)

Calcium (Tricalcium Phosphate)
- Balance Complete™ 40%

Calcium Sulfate
- AlkaLime 15% DV (201 mg)

Chloride
- Mineral Essence™ 3 g/serving

Chromium
- Master Formula™ 100% DV (120 mcg)
- Balance Complete™ 30%

Copper
- Master Formula™ 20% DV (350 mcg)
- ImmuPro™ 18% DV (0.16 mg)
- JuvaTone® 80% DV (1.6 mg)

Fluorine
- Mineral Essence™ ionic trace amounts

Iodine
- Balance Complete™ 25%
- NingXia NITRO® 75 µg (DV 50%)
- Slique® Shake 25%

Iodine from Kelp
- Thyromin™ 365% (547 mcg)
- MulitGreens™
- Master Formula™

Iron
- Master Formula™ 60% DV (10 mg)
- Mineral Essence™ ionic trace amounts
- ICP™ 1mg/serving
- JuvaPower® 10% DV (1.7 mg)
- MultiGreens™ 4% DV (0.8 mg)
- Slique® Bar Tropical Bar 4%
- NingXia Red® 2% (0.4 mg)
- Balance Complete™ 2%

Lithium
- Mineral Essence™ ionic trace amounts

Magnesium
- Master Formula™ 15% DV (60 mg)
- Mineral Essence™ 350mg/serving
- Super B™ 2% DV (10 mg)
- Super Cal™ Plus 119 mg
- KidScents® MightyVites™ 4.5 mg
- Balance Complete™ 35%

Magnesium Bisglycinate
- PowerGize™ 20 mg
- Super B™ 10 mg

Magnesium Carbonate
- FemiGen™ 2% DV (5 mg)
- MegCal 61% DV (245 mg)
- Thyromin™

Magnesium Citrate
- AminoWise™ 277 mg
- MegaCal™ 61% DV (245 mg)
- Super Cal™ Plus 119 mg

Magnesium Oxide
- Balance Complete™

Magnesium Phosphate
- AlkaLime

Magnesium Stearate (tablet lubricator)
- BLM™
- Detoxzyme®
- Essentialzymes-4™
- ImmuPro™
- Sulfurzyme Capsules
- Thyromin™
- JuvaTone®
- KidScents® MightyVites™
- KidScents® MightyZyme™
- Super C™ Chewable
- Master Formula™

Magnesium Sulfate
- MegaCal™ 61% DV (245 mg)

Manganese
- Master Formula™ 100% DV (2 mg)
- Super B™ 25% DV (0.5 mg)

Manganese Citrate
- BLM™ 715 mg

NOTES:

NOTES:

Manganese Sulfate
- Super C™ Tablets 90% DV (2 mg)
- Mega Cal 16% DV (320 mcg)

Methylsulfonylmethane (MSM or sulfur)
- BLM™
- Sulfurzyme® Capsules
- Sulfurzyme® Powder

Molybdenum
- Master Formula™ 100% DV (75 mcg)
- Balance Complete™ 20%

Phosphorus
- Balance Complete™ 25%

Piperine
- AgilEase

Potassium
- Master Formula™
- Super C™ Tablets <1% DV (20 mg)
- Balance Complete™ 9% DV (330mg)

Potassium Bicarbonate
- AlkaLime® 22% DV (505 mg)

Potassium Chloride
- AlkaLime® 2% DV (95 mg)
- Master Formula™ <2% (50mg)
- Super C™ tablets

Potassium Citrate
- AminoWise™ 277 mg
- Thyromin™

Potassium Phosphate
- AlkaLime® 2% DV (95 mg)

Potassium Sulfate
- AlkaLime® 2% DV (95 mg)

Selenium
- Balance Complete™ 30%

Selenium (amino acid)
- Master Formula™ 110% DV (75 mcg)
- Mineral Essence™ ionic trace amounts
- Super B™ 70% DV (50 mcg)
- Balance Complete™ 30%
- CardioGize™ 180% DV (100 mcg)
- ImmuPro™ 124% DV (68 mcg)
- KidScents® MightyVites™ 4.5 mcg

Silicon
- Master Formula™
- Mineral Essence™ ionic trace amounts
- ComforTone®

Sodium
- Mineral Essence™ 10mg/serving
- Balance Complete™ 5% (115 mg)
- Pure Protein™ Complete 10% DV (240 mg)
- JuvaPower® 1% DV (25 mg)
- Juva Tone <1% DV (16 mg)
- MultiGreens™ <1% DV (8 mg)
- Slique® Bar Berry 3% DV (70 mg)
- NingXia Red® 2% (35 mg)

Sodium Bicarbonate
- AlkaLime® 22% DV (505 mg)

Sodium Chloride
- Pure Protein™ Complete

Sodium Citrate
- AminoWise™ 2.77 mg

Sodium Hyaluronate
- AgilEase™

Sodium Phosphate
- AlkaLime® 22% DV (505 mg)

Sodium Sulfate
- AlkaLime® 22% DV (505 mg)

Sulfur
- Mineral Essence™ ionic trace amounts
- BLM™ (as MSM)
- Sulfurzyme® Capsules (as MSM)
- Sulfurzyme® Powder (as MSM)

Thallium
- Mineral Essence™ ionic trace amounts

Zinc
- Master Formula™ 100% DV (15 mg)
- Mineral Essence™ ionic trace amounts
- Super B™ 20% DV (3 mg)
- Super C™ Tablets 10% DV (1 mg)
- Balance Complete™ 25%
- Pure Protein™ Complete 100% DV (15 mg)
- KidScents® MightyVites™ 0.9 mg

NOTES:

NOTES:

DIGESTIVE ENZYMES

Amylase
Breaks down starch, breads, and pasta
- Pure Protein™ Complete (Alpha and Beta)
- Essentialzymes-4™
- Allerzyme™
- Detoxzyme®
- KidScents® MightyZyme™
- EndoGize™ 448 mg
- Balance Complete™
- Slique® CitriSlim™

Alpha-galactosidase
Breaks down polysaccharides, beans, and veggies (gas)
- Allerzyme™
- Detoxzyme®

Betaine HCL (Betaine hydrochloride)
Promotes the production of hydrochloric acid to aid digestion. Helps the body absorb B12, Calcium, Iron, and Proteins.
- Essentialzyme™
- FemiGen™

Bromelain
Breaks down peptides and amino acids found in meat, dairy, eggs, and grains, as well as seeds, nuts, and leafy greens.
- Pure Protein™ Complete 50% DV (0.75 mg)
- Essentialzyme™
- Essentialzymes-4™
- Allerzyme™
- Detoxzyme®
- KidScents® MightyZyme™
- Balance Complete™

Cellulase
Breaks down man-made fiber, plant fiber, fruits, and veggies.
- Pure Protein™ Complete 50% DV (0.75 mg)
- Essentialzymes-4™
- Allerzyme™
- Detoxzyme®
- EndoGize™ 448 mg
- KidScents® MightyZyme™ 81 mg
- Slique® CitriSlim™

Diastase (barley malt)
Breaks down grain sugars and starch.
- Allerzyme™

Glucoamylase
Breaks down starchy foods and cereals.
Flushes the body of dead white blood cells.
- Detoxzyme®
- EndoGize™ 448 mg

Invertase
Breaks down sugar found in sweets and deserts.
Breaks connection between fructose and glucose.
- Allerzyme™
- Detoxzyme®

Lactase
Breaks down lactose (dairy sugars).
- Allerzyme™
- Detoxzyme®
- Pure Protein™ Complete 50% DV (0.75 mg)
- Balance Complete™

Lipase
Breaks down dietary fats and oils.
Helps liver function.
- Pure Protein™ Complete 50% DV (0.75 mg)
- Essentialzymes-4™
- Allerzyme™
- Detoxzyme®
- KidScents® MightyZyme™
- ICP™ 123 mg
- Balance Complete™
- Slique® CitriSlim™

Pancrelipase (extract from pig pancreatic glands)
Combo of lipase, protease, and amylase usually created by the pancreas. Good for those with poorly performing pancreases.
- Essentialzyme™

Pancreatin (pancreas from pigs or cows)
Helps produce other enzymes: amylase, lipase, and protease. Good for those with poorly performing pancreases.
- Essentialzyme™
- Essentialzymes-4™

NOTES:

NOTES:

Papain
Digestive aid. May help with parasites, psoriasis, shingles, diarrhea, and runny nose.
- Pure Protein™ Complete 50% DV (0.75 mg)
- Essentialzyme™
- Essentialzymes-4™
- Balance Complete™

Peptidase
Finishes breaking down proteases. Helps support immunity and inflammation.
- Allerzyme™
- KidScents® MightyZyme™
- Essentialzymes-4™ 186 mg
- ICP™ 123 mg

Phytase
Helps with bone health and minerals.
- Essentialzymes-4™
- Allerzyme™
- Detoxzyme®
- KidScents® MightyZyme™
- ICP™ 123 mg

Protease 3.0
Supports circulation and toxicity. Higher acid content breaks down animal protein.
- Essentialzymes-4™ 186 mg
- ICP™ 123 mg
- KidScents® MightyZyme™ 81 mg

Protease 4.5
Lower acidic content.
- Essentialzymes-4™ 186 mg
- ICP™ 123 mg
- KidScents MightyZyme™ 81 mg

Protease 6.0
Carries away toxins in the blood. Least acidic.
- Pure Protein™ Complete 50% DV (0.75 mg)
- Essentialzymes-4™
- Allerzyme™
- Detoxzyme®
- KidScents® MightyZyme™
- ICP™ 123 mg
- Slique® CitriSlim™

Trypsin
Breaks down proteins. For muscle growth and hormone production.
- Essentialzyme™

AMINO ACIDS

Amino Acids (general)
- Mineral Essence™
- NingXia Red®
- AminoWise™

B-alanine
- AminoWise™ 5.7 mg

L-alpha glycerylphosphorylcholine
- MindWise™ 378.4 mg

L-a-phosphatidylserine
- CortiStop®

L-a-phosphatidylcholine
- CortiStop®

L-arginine
- AminoWise™ 5.7 mg
- EndoGize™ 448 mg
- Super Cal™ Plus
- MultiGreens™ 1.5 g

L-carnitine
- FemiGen™ 1.2 g

L-citrulline
- AminoWise™ 5.7 mg

L-cysteine
- Thyromin™ 439.7 mg
- MultiGreens™ 1.5 g

L-cysteine HCL (hydrochloride)
- FemiGen™ 1.2 g
- Thyromin™ 439.7 mg
- JuvaTone® 3.3 g

L-glutamine
- AminoWise™ 5.7 mg
- Pure Protein™ Complete

NOTES:

NOTES:

L-isoleucine
- Pure Protein™ Complete

L-leucine
- Pure Protein™ Complete

L-lysine
- Pure Protein
- Super Cal™ Plus

L-methionine
- Pure Protein™ Complete

L-phenylalanine
- FemiGen™ 1.2 g

L-taurine
- AminoWise™ 5.7 mg
- JuvaPower® 7.5 g

L-tyrosine
- Thyromin™ 439.7 mg
- MultiGreens™ 1.5 g

L-valine
- Pure Protein™ Complete

Selenium (amino acid)
- Master Formula™ 110% DV (75 mcg)
- Mineral Essence™ trace amounts
- Super B™ 70% DV (50 mcg)
- Balance Complete™ 30%
- CardioGize™ 180% DV (100 mcg)
- ImmuPro™ 124% DV (68 mcg)
- KidScents® MightyVites™ 4.5 mcg

PREBIOTICS

Prebiotics (Wolfberry Fiber)
- Master Formula™
- Sulfurzyme® Powder
- Sulfurzyme® Capsules
- MightyPro™
- NingXia Red®

Prebiotics (fructo-oligosaccharides FCOs)
- AminoWise™
- Sulfurzyme Powder 2.02 g
- KidScents® MightyPro™
- Master Formula™ 208 mg

PROBIOTICS

Probiotics
- Life 9™
- MightyPro™
- Pure Protein™ Complete

Lactobacillus acidophilus
- Pure Protein™ Complete 50% DV (0.75 mg)

Probiotics in Life 9™
1. *Lactobacillus acidophilus*
2. *Lactobacillus plantarum*
3. *Lactobacillus rhamnosus*
4. *Lactobacillus salivarius*
5. *Streptococcus thermophiles*
6. *Bifidobacterium breve*
7. *Bifidobacterium bifidum*
8. *Bifidobacterium longum*
9. *Bifidobacterium lactis*

Probiotics in MightyPro™
1. *Lactobacillus acidophilus* (also in Pure Protein™ Complete)
2. *Lactobacillus plantarum*
3. *Lactobacillus rhamnosus*
4. *Streptococcus thermophilus*
5. *Lactobacillus rhamnosus*
6. *Lactobacillus paracasei*
7. *Bifidobacterium infantis*

NOTES:

NOTES:

NUTRIENTS, HERBS, & OTHER INGREDIENTS

Acai Puree
- MindWise™

Acerola Cherry Powder
- Super C™ Chewable

Acerola Fruit Extract
- Super C™ Chewable 460 mg
- Master Formula™ 100 mg

Acetyl-L-Carnitine
- MindWise™ 378.4 mg

Acid Stable Protease
- EndoGize™ 448 mg
-

Adrenal Powder
- Thyromin™ 439.7 mg

Alfalfa Leaf Powder
- Essentialzyme
- MultiGreens™ 1.5 g

Alfalfa Sprout Powder
- Essentialzyme
- JuvaTone® 3.3 g
- KidScents® MightZyme 81 mg

Aloe Vera Leaf Extract
- ICP™ 5.6 g
- JuvaPower® 7.5 g
- Balance Complete™

Amla Fruit Extract
- KidScents® MightyVites™

American Ginseng Root
- FemiGen™ 1.2 g

Anise Fruit Oil
- ParaFree™ 2250 mg

Anise Seed
- JuvaPower® 7.5 g

Annatto
- KidScents® MightyVites 97 mg

Apple Fruit Skin Extract
- Master Formula™ 100 mg

Apple Juice Powder
- KidScents® MightyZyme™

Apple Pectin
- ComforTone® 694 mg

Arabinogalactan
- ImmuPro™ 940 mg

Aronia Juice Concentrate
- NingXia Red® 58 g

Ashwagandha Root Powder
- EndoGize™ 448 mg
- PowerGize™

Astragalus Root Powder
- CardioGize™

Atlantic Kelp
- Master Formula™ 42 mg

B-alanine
- AminoWise™ 5.7 mg

Barberry Bark
- ComforTone® 694 mg

Barley Grass
- Allerzyme™
- MultiGreens™ 1.5 g
- KidScents® MightyVites™ 97 mg
- Balance Complete™
- Master Formula™ 42 mg

Barley Sprouted Seed
- JuvaPower® 7.5 g

NOTES:

NOTES:

Basil Leaf Concentrate
- Master Formula™ 100 mg

Bee Pollen
- Essentialzymes-4™
- MultiGreens™ 1.5 g

Bee Propolis
- JuvaTone® 3.3 g

Beet Root Powder
- JuvaPower® 7.5 g
- JuvaTone® 3.3 g
- KidScents® MightyVites™ 97 mg

Bentonite
- ComforTone® 694 mg

Beta-Carotene
- Balance Complete™

Bilberry Fruit Extract
- Master Formula™ 100 mg

Black Cohosh Root Extract
- CortiStop®
- FemiGen™ 1.2 g

Black Currant Fruit Extract
- Master Formula™ 100 mg

Blackberry Fruit Concentrate
- Master Formula™ 100 mg

Blackberry Juice Concentrate
- NingXia Zyng™

Blueberry Fruit Concentrate
- Master Formula™ 100 mg

Blueberry Juice Concentrate
- NingXia Red® 58 g

Boron Citrate
- Master Formula™ 42 mg

Branched Chain Amino Acids
- AminoWise™ 5.7 mg

Broccoli Floret/Stem Concentrate
- Master Formula™ 100 mg

Broccoli Floret/Stalk Powder
- JuvaPower® 7.5 g
- KidScents® MightyVites™ 97 mg

Broccoli Seed Concentrate
- Master Formula™ 100 mg

Brown Rice Bran
- Balance Complete™

Brussels Sprout Head Concentrate
- Master Formula™ 100 mg

Buckthorn Bark
- Rehemogen™ 3 ml

Burdock Root
- ComforTone® 694 mg
- Rehemogen™ 3 ml

Cabbage Palm Concentrate
- Master Formula™ 100 mg

Cactus Cladode Powder
- CardioGize™

Calcium Silicate (anti-caking agent)
- AminoWise™
- Sulfurzyme™ Powder

Camellia Sinensis Leaf Extract
- Master Formula™ 100 mg

Camu Camu Whole Fruit Powder
- Super C™ Chewable 460 mg
- Master Formula™ 100 mg

Cane Sugar
- Pure Protein™ Complete
- NingXia Zyng™

NOTES:

NOTES:

Carbonated Water
- NingXia Zyng™

Caraway Fruit Oil
- Digest & Cleanse™ 710 mg

Cardamom Seed Powder
- CardioGize™

Carrageenan
- SleepEssence™

Carrot Root Concentrate
- Master Formula™ 100 mg

Carrot Root Powder
- Essentialzyme™
- KidScents MightyZyme™ 81 mg

Cascara Sagrada Bark
- ComforTone® 694 mg
- Rehemogen™ 3 ml

Cassia Branch/Stem Concentrate
- Master Formula™ 100 mg

Cat's Claw Bark Powder
- CardioGize™

Cayenne Fruit
- ComforTone® 694 mg
- Super C™ Tablet 78 mg

Cellulose
- ICP™ 5.6 g
- JuvaTone®

Cellulose Film-Coating
- JuvaTone®

Cherry Juice Concentrate
- NingXia Red® 58 g

Chicory Root
- Balance Complete™

Chokeberry Fruit Concentrate
- Master Formula™ 100 mg

Choline
- Juva Tone 3.3 g
- MultiGreens™ 1.5 g
- NingXia NITRO®
- Master Formula™ 208 mg

Chromium Amino Nicotinate
- Balance Complete™

Cinnamon Bark
- Balance Complete™

Citric Acid
- AlkaLime®
- AminoWise™
- MindWise™
- KidScents® MightyPro™
- NingXia Zyng™

Citrus Bioflavonoids
- Super C™ Chewable 460 mg
- Super C™ Tablet 78 mg
- Master Formula™ 42 mg

Citrus Flavonoids
- KidScents® MightyVites™ 97 mg

Clove Bud
- K & B™ 3 ml

Cocoa Powder
- Pure Protein™ Complete

Coconut Fruit Oil
- SleepEssence™
- Digest & Cleanse™ 710 mg
- Inner Defense™ 405 mg
- Longevity™ 720 mg

Coconut Nectar
- NingXia NITRO®

Coffea Arabica Fruit Extract
- Master Formula™ 100 mg

NOTES:

NOTES:

Cramp Bark
- FemiGen™ 1.2 g

Collards Leaf Concentrate
- Master Formula™ 100 mg

CoQ10 (ubiquinone) Fat Soluble
- OmegaGize3™
- CardioGize™
- MindWise™ 378.4 mg

Croscarmellose Sodium
- Master Formula™

Cucumber Fruit Powder
- JuvaPower® 7.5 g

Cumin Seed Powder
- Detoxzyme®
- Essentialzyme™

Cumin Seed Oil
- ParaFree™ 2250 mg

Curcuminoids Complex Rhizome Extract (Turmeric) Fat Soluble
- AgilEase™ (537.5 mg)

D-Alpha-Tocopherol Acetate
- NingXia Zyng™

D-Ribose
- NingXia NITRO®

DHEA (derived from wild yam)
- CortiStop®
- EndoGize™ 448 mg
- PD 80/20™ 500 mg

Damiana Leaf
- FemiGen™ 1.2 g

Dandelion Root Extract
- K & B™ 3 ml
- JuvaTone® 3.3 g

Desert Hyacinth Root Powder
- PowerGize™

Dextrates
- KidScents® MightyZyme™

Dextrose
- ImmuPro™

D-Calcium Pantothenate
- NingXia Zyng™

DI-Methionine
- JuvaTone® 3.3 g

Dill Seed
- JuvaPower® 7.5 g

Dimethylgycine HCL
- FemiGen™ 1.2 g

Distilled Water (see also Water)
- Rehemogen™

Dong Quai Root Powder
- CardioGize™
- FemiGen™ 1.2 g

Echinacea Root
- ComforTone® 694 mg
- JuvaTone® 3.3 g

Eleuthero Root
- MultiGreens™ 1.5 g

Epimedium Aerial Parts
- EndoGize™ 448 mg
- FemiGen™ 1.2 g

Epimedium Leaf Powder
- PowerGize™

Erythritol
- KidScents® MightyPro™

NOTES:

NOTES:

Ethanol Alcohol
- K & B™
- Rehemogen™

European Elder Fruit Concentrate
- Master Formula™ 100 mg

Fennel Fruit
- K & B™ 3 ml

Fennel Seed
- ComforTone® 694 mg
- ICP™ 5.6 g
- JuvaPower® 7.5 g

Fenugreek Seed Extract
- PowerGize™

Fermented Polysaccharide Complex
- Super Cal™ Plus

Fiber
- ICP™ 2g/serving

Fish (Basa)
- OmegaGize3™

Fish (tilapia, carp)
- ParaFree™
- Inner Defense™

Fish Gelatin
- ParaFree™
- Inner Defense™ 405 mg

Flax Seed Powder
- ICP™ 5.6 g
- JuvaPower® 7.5 g

Fractionated Coconut Oil
- MegaCal™
- Digest & Cleanse™ 710 mg
- Longevity 720 mg

Fructooligosaccharides
- AminoWise™
- Sulfurzyme Powder 2.02 g
- KidScents® MightyPro™
- Master Formula™ 208 mg

Fructose
- Balance Complete™

Garlic Bulb Extract
- CardioGize™
- ComforTone® 694 mg

Garlic Clove Concentrate
- Master Formula™ 100 mg

Gelatin
- BLM™
- CortiStop®
- Essentialzymes-4™
- PD 80/20™
- Super Cal™ Plus
- Thyromin™
- ComforTone®
- MultiGreens™
- OmegaGize3™

Geranium Aerial Parts
- K & B™ 3 ml

German Chamomile Flower Extract
- K & B™ 3 ml
- ComforTone® 694 mg

Ginger Root
- ComforTone® 694 mg
- JuvaPower® 7.5 g

Glucosamine Sulfate
- BLM™ (from shellfish)
- AgilEase™ (not from shellfish)

Glycerin
- MindWise™
- SleepEssence™
- ParaFree™
- Inner Defense™

Grape Seed Extract
- NingXia Red® 100 mg

NOTES:

NOTES:

Grapefruit Whole Fruit Powder
- Master Formula™ 42 mg

Green Tea Extract
- NingXia NITRO®

Guar Gum
- Master Formula™

Guar Gum Seed Powder
- ICP™ 5.6 g
- Balance Complete™

Guava Fruit Extract
- KidScents® MightyVites™ 97 mg

HPMC Targeted Release Capsule
- Life 9™

Hawthorn Berry Powder
- CardioGize™

Holy Basil Aerial Parts Extract
- KidScents® MightyVites™

Honey
- Mineral Essence™ 5 ml

Hops Flower Extract
- Super Cal™ Plus

Hydroxypropyl Cellulose
- ImmuPro™
- Super C™ Chewable

Hypromellose
- Allerzyme™
- CardioGize™
- Detoxzyme®
- Essentialzymes-4™
- PowerGize™
- Sulfurzyme™ Capsules
- Digest & Cleanse™
- Longevity™
- Master Formula™

Inositol
- JuvaTone® 3.3 g

Japanese Sophora Flower Extract
- Master Formula™ 100 mg

Juniper Branch/Leaf/Fruit
- K & B™ 3 ml

Juniper Berry Extract
- K & B™ 3ml

Kelp Whole Thallus
- MultiGreens™ 1.5 g

Konjac
- Balance Complete™

Korean Ginseng Extract
- NingXia NITRO®

Lecithin
- SleepEssence™
- Balance Complete™

Lemon Peel Extract
- KidScents® MightyVites™ 97 mg

Lemon Rind
- MegaCal™ 2.8 g

Licorice Root Extract
- FemiGen™ 1.2 mg
- Rehemogen™ 3 ml

Lime Fruit Powder
- AminoWise™ 1.2 mg
- Master Formula™ 42 mg

Longjack Root Extract
- EndoGize™ 448 mg
- PowerGize™

Luo han guo Fruit Extract
- MindWise™
- Pure Protein
- Balance Complete™

Lycopene
- Master Formula™ 42 mg

MCT
- Balance Complete™

NOTES:

NOTES:

Maitake Mushroom Mycelia Powder
- ImmuPro™ 940 mg

Malic Acid
- MindWise™
- KidScents® MightyVites™
- NingXia Red®

Maltodextrin
- ImmuPro™
- Master Formula™

Mangosteen Fruit Concentrate
- Master Formula™ 100 mg

Marine Minerals
- Super Cal™ Plus

Microcrystalline Cellulose
- KidScents® MightyZyme™
- Life 9™
- Master Formula™

Mixed Carotenoids
- OmegaGize3™
- Balance Complete™

Mixed Tocopherols
- Longevity™
- Balance Complete™

Modified Cornstarch
- SleepEssence™

Mojave Yucca Root
- ICP™ 5.6 g

Motherwort Herb Powder
- CardioGize™

Muira Puama Bark
- EndoGize™ 448 mg
- FemiGen™ 1.2 g
- PowerGize™

Mulberry Leaf Extract
- NingXia NITRO®

Mushroom Mycelia Powder
- ImmuPro™ 940 mg

Natural Flavors
- AminoWise™
- MindWise™
- Pure Protein™ Complete
- NingXia NITRO®
- NingXia Zyng™
- Balance Complete™

Natural Fruit Punch Flavor
- KidScents® MightPro™

Natural Mixed Berry Flavor
- KidScents® MightyZyme™

Natural Sweetener
- KidScents® MightyVites™

Neohesperidin Derivative
- Balance Complete™

Niacinamide
- NingXia Zyng™

NingXia Wolfberry Fruit Powder
- AminoWise™ 1.2 mg
- Sulfurzyme™ Capsules 1.8 g
- Sulfurzyme™ Powder 2.02 g
- KidScents® MightyPro™

NingXia Wolfberry Puree
- NingXia Red® 58 g

Non-GMO Cornstarch
- Super Cal™ Plus

Nitro Juice Blend Concentrate
(cherry, kiwi, blueberry, acerola, billberry, black currant, raspberry, strawberry, cranberry)
- NingXia NITRO®

Nonfat Dry Milk
- Balance Complete™

Non-GMO Tapioca Dextrose
- Super C™ Chewable

Oat Bran Powder
- ICP™ 5.6 g
- JuvaPower® 7.5 g

NOTES:

NOTES:

Olive Fruit Oil
- ParaFree™ 2250 mg
- Master Formula™ 42 mg

Omega-3 Fatty Acids
- OmegaGize3™ 445 mg

Onion Bulb Extract
- Master Formula™ 100 mg

Orange Fruit Juice Powder
- KidScents® MightyVites™ 97 mg

Orange Whole Fruit Powder
- Master Formula™ 42 mg

Oregano Leaf Concentrate
- Master Formula™ 100 mg

Oregon Grape Root
- JuvaTone® 3.3 g
- Rehemogen™ 3 ml

Organic Ground Nutmeg
- Pure Protein Vanilla Spice only

Orgen-kid Leaf Extract
- KidScents® MightyVites™ 97 mg

PABA
- Master Formula™ 42 mg
- Super B™

Palm Olein
- Master Formula™

Parsley Leaf Extract
- K & B™ 3 ml
- Thyromin™ 439.7 mg
- JuvaTone® 3.3 g

Peach Bark
- Rehemogen™ 3 ml

Pear Juice Concentrate
- NingXia Zyng™

Pectin
- NingXia Red®
- NingXia NITRO®

Pituitary Powder
- Thyromin™ 439.7 mg

Plantain Leaf
- Allerzyme™

Plum Juice Concentrate
- NingXia Red® 58 g

Poke Root
- Rehemogen™ 3 ml

Polyphenols Extract
- AminoWise™ 1.2 mg

Pomegranate Fruit Extract
- MindWise™ 378.4 mg

Pomegranate Juice Concentrate
- MindWise™
- NingXia Red® 58 g

Porcine Gelatin
- Prostate Health™

Pregnenolone
- CortiStop®
- PD 80/20™ 500 mg

Prickly Ash Bark
- Rehemogen™ 3 ml

Proprietary V-Fiber Blend
- Balance Complete™

Psyllium Seed
- ComforTone® 694 mg
- ICP™ 5.6 g
- JuvaPower® 7.5 g

Pumpkin Seed Oil
- Prostate Health™ 175 mg

Pure Vanilla Extract
- NingXia Red®

Purified Water (see also Water)
- OmegaGize3™
- NingXia NITRO®

NOTES:

NOTES:

Pyridoxine Hydrochloride
- NingXia Zyng™
- Pure Protein™ Complete

Raspberry Fruit Concentrate
- Master Formula™ 100 mg

Raspberry Fruit Powder
- ImmuPro™ 940 mg

Red Clover Blossom
- Rehemogen™ 3 ml

Reishi Whole Mushroom Powder
- ImmuPro™ 940 mg

Retinyl Palmitate
- NingXia Zyng™

Rhododendron Leaf Extract
- MindWise™ 378.4 mg

Rice Bran
- Detoxzyme®
- ICP™ 5.6 g
- JuvaPower® 7.5 g
- OmegaGize3™

Rice Flour
- BLM™
- CortiStop®
- Essentialzymes-4™
- PD 80/20™
- PowerGize™
- Sulfurzyme™ Capsules

Roman Chamomile Aerial Parts
- K & B™ 3 ml

Rose Hips Fruit Powder
- Super C™ Chewable 460 mg

Royal Jelly
- K & B™ 3 ml
- Rehemogen™ 3 ml
- Mineral Essence™ 5 ml

Rutin Flower Bud Powder
- Super C™ Tablet 78 mg

Sage Aerial Parts
- K & B™ 3 ml

Salt
- Mineral Essence™ 5 ml

Sarsaparilla Root
- Rehemogen™ 3 ml

Saw Palmetto Fruit Extract
- Prostate Health™ 235 mg

Selenium
- Balance Complete™

Sesame Seed Oil
- ParaFree™ 2250 mg

Sesbania Leaf Extract
- KidScents® MightyVites™

Shellfish (crab and shrimp)
- BLM™

Silica
- Allerzyme™
- AminoWise™
- CardioGize™
- CortiStop®
- Detoxzyme®
- Prostate Health™
- Sulfurzyme™ Capsules
- Digest & Cleanse™
- MultiGreens™
- KidScents® MightyVites™
- KidScents® MightyZyme™
- Life 9™
- Longevity

Silicon Dioxide
- BLM™
- Essentialzymes-4™
- ImmuPro™
- PowerGize™
- ComforTone®
- JuvaTone®
- OmegaGize3™
- Super C™ Chewable
- Master Formula™

NOTES:

NOTES:

Slippery Elm Bark
- JuvaPower® 7.5 g

Sorbitol
- SleepEssence™
- KidScents® MightyZyme™
- Super C™ Chewable

Soy
- CortiStop®
- EndoGize™ 448 mg

Spinach Leaf Concentrate
- Master Formula™ 100 mg

Spinach Leaf Powder
- JuvaPower® 7.5 g

Spirulina
- MultiGreens™ 1.5 g

Squaw Vine Aerial Parts
- FemiGen™ 1.2 g

Stearic Acid
- Super Cal™ Plus
- KidScents® MightyZyme™
- Super C™ Chewable
- Master Formula™

Stevia
- AlkaLime
- AminoWise™
- ImmuPro™
- Pure Protein
- Sulfurzyme Powder
- KidScents® MightyVites™
- KidScents® MightyZyme™
- Super C™ Chewable
- NingXia Red®
- NingXia Zyng™

Stillingia Root
- Rehemogen™ 3 ml

Strawberry Fruit Powder
- ImmuPro™ 940 mg
- KidScents® MightyVites™ 97 mg

Sunflower Lecithin
- MindWise™
- Master Formula™

Sweet Cherry Fruit Concentrate
- Master Formula™ 100 mg

Tomato Fruit Concentrate
- Master Formula™ 100 mg

Tangerine Whole Fruit Powder
- Master Formula™ 42 mg

Tapioca Maltodextrin
- AminoWise™

Tapioca Starch
- AminoWise™

Tartaric Acid
- AlkaLime®
- NingXia Red®

Tea Leaf Extract
- Super Cal™ Plus

Thyme Leaf Powder
- Essentialzyme™

Thyroid Powder
- Thyromin™ 439.7 mg

Tomato Fruit Flakes
- JuvaPower® 7.5 g

Tree Nuts(coconut)
- Inner Defense™
- Digest & Cleanse™
- Longevity™

Tribulus Fruit Extract
- EndoGize™ 448 mg
- PowerGize™

Turmeric Root Concentrate
- Master Formula™ 100 mg

Turmeric Root Oil
- Master Formula™

NOTES:

NOTES:

Turmeric Root Powder
- MindWise™ 378.4 mg
- AgilEase™ 537.5 mg

Type II Collagen
- AgilEase™
- AgilEase™
- BLM™

Uva-ursi Leaf Extract
- K & B™ 3 ml

Water
- Allerzyme™
- CardioGize™
- Detoxzyme®
- K & B™
- MindWise™
- Prostate Health™
- SleepEssence™
- ComforTone®
- Digest & Cleanse™
- ParaFree™
- Inner Defense™
- Longevity

Whey Protein Concentrate
- Balance Complete™

White Tea Leaf Extract
- NingXia Zyng™

Wild Yam Root (see also DHEA)
- FemiGen™ 1.2 g

Winged Treebine Root Extract
- Super Cal™ Plus

Wolfberry Fruit Polysaccharide
- ImmuPro™ 940 mg

Wolfberry Fruit Powder
- KidScents® MightyVites™ 97 mg

Wolfberry Puree
- NingXia Zyng™

Wolfberry Seed Oil
- NingXia NITRO®

Xanthan Gum
- Pure Protein™ Complete
- NingXia NITRO
- Balance Complete™

Xylitol
- MegaCal™ 2.8 g
- KidScents® MightPro
- Balance Complete™

Zinc water (Zinc Aspartate)
- EndoGize™ 20% DV (2 mg)

Zinc (Zinc Bisglycinate)
- ImmuPro™ 45% DV (5 mg)

Zinc (Zinc Gluconate)
- AminoWise™ 1.2 mg
- MegaCal™ 2% DV (260 mcg)
- Super C™ tablets

Zinc (Zinc Glycinate Chelate)
- PowerGize™ 5 mg

Zinc Oxide
- Balance Complete™

NOTES:

NOTES:

ALLERGY AND SPECIAL NOTES LIST

This list is not exhaustive. Please check with Young Living® Product Support for specific inquiries. Products are reformulated all the time. This may not be a fully up-to-date list at the time you are reading it.

SUPPLEMENTS WITHOUT ESSENTIAL OILS
- Life 9™
- KidScents® MightyPro™
- KidScents® MightyVites™
- Sulfurzyme® Capsules
- Sulfurzyme® Powder
- PD 80/20™

SUPPLEMENTS THAT ARE MOSTLY ESSENTIAL OILS
- Digest & Cleanse™
- Inner Defense™
- Longevity™
- SleepEssence™
- ParaFree™
- Prostate Health™
- Slique® CitriSlim™ liquid capsule
- Master Formula™ liquid capsule (about half)

SUPPLEMENTS THAT CONTAIN CORN
- AlkaLime®
- Allerzyme
- Slique® Gum
- Slique® Shake

SUPPLEMENTS THAT CONTAIN DAIRY
- Allerzyme™
- Balance Complete™
- Pure Protein™ Complete
- NingXia NITRO®
- Super C™ Chewables

SUPPLEMENTS THAT CONTAIN GLUTEN (POTENTIAL)

Barley Grass *(cross-contamination may occur)*
- Allerzyme™
- MultiGreens™ 1.5 g
- KidScents® MightyVites™ 97 mg
- Balance Complete™
- Master Formula™ 42 mg

Barley Sprouted Seed *(cross-contamination may occur)*
- JuvaPower® 7.5 g

SUPPLEMENTS THAT CONTAIN NUTS
- Slique® Bars (actual nuts)

Coconut and derivatives of coconut
- MindWise™
- Slique® CitriSlim™
- Inner Defense™
- Digest & Cleanse™
- SleepEssence™
- Longevity™

SUPPLEMENTS THAT CONTAIN SHELLFISH

Glucosamine sulfate in the form ground up shrimp bodies
- BLM™
- *Note: AgilEase™ contains Glucosamine sulfate that is not sourced from shellfish.*

SUPPLEMENTS THAT ARE NOT VEGAN
- Allerzyme™
- BLM™
- Inner Defense™
- Longevity™
- Master Formula™
- MultiGreens™
- OmegaGize3™
- Prostate Health™
- Pure Protein™ Complete
- Slique Bars
- Super C™
- Super Cal™ Plus
- Thyromin™

DIGESTIVE ENZYME USAGE GUIDE

	ESSENTIALZYMES-4™	ESSENTIALZYME™	ALLERZYME™	DETOXZYME®	MIGHTYZYME™	ENDOGIZE™ (HORMONES & ENZYMES)	ICP™ (COLON & ENZYMES)
AMYLASE Breaks down starches, breads, and pastas.	√		√	√	√	√	
ALPHA-GALACTOSIDASE Breaks down foods that cause gas.			√	√			
BROMELAIN Breaks down protein and grains. Supports blood to help with inflammation.	√	√	√	√	√		
CELLULASE Breaks down man-made fiber, plant fiber, fruits, and veggies.	√		√	√	√	√	
DIASTASE (contains barley malt) Breaks down grain sugars and starch.			√				
GLUCOAMYLASE Breaks down starchy foods and cereals. Flushes body of dead white blood cells.				√		√	
INVERTASE Breaks down table sugar. Breaks the connection between fructose and glucose.			√	√			
LACTASE Breaks down dairy sugars. Helps with lactose intolerance.			√	√			
LIPASE Dietary fats and oils. Helps liver function.			√	√	√		√
PEPTIDASE Finishes breaking down Proteases. Supports the immunity and inflammation.				√	√		√
PHYTASE Helps with bone health. Pulls needed minerals from grains.	√		√	√	√		√
PROTEASE 3.0 Supports blood circulation and toxicity. Breaks down animal protein.	√				√		√
PROTEASE 4.5 Helps with sinusitis. Has a lower acidity.	√				√		√
PROTEASE 6.0 Helps carry away toxins. Helps reduce pain and varicose veins. Least acidic.	√		√	√	√		√
PAPAIN Digestive aid, and may help with parasites, psoriasis, shingles, diarrhea, and sniffles.	√	√					
BETAINE HCL (Betaine hydrochloride) Promotes hydrochloric acid to help digestion. Helps absorb B12, Calcium, Iron, and Proteins.		√					
PANCREALIPASE (pancreas gland extract from pig) Combo of Lipase, Protease, and Amylase. Supports a poorly performing pancreas.		√					
PANCREATIN (pancreas from pigs or cows) Helps produce amylase, lipase, and protease. Supports a poorly performing pancreas.	√	√					
TRYPSIN Breaks down proteins. For muscle growth and hormone production.		√					

HORMONE SUPPORT USAGE GUIDE

	FEMIGEN™	PD 80/20™	CORTISTOP™	ENDOGIZE™	THYROMIN™
ADRENAL FATIGUE				✓	
APPETITE CONTROL	✓				
ANIMAL GLAND EXTRACT - ADRENAL					✓
ANIMAL GLAND EXTRACT - PITUITARY					✓
ANIMAL GLAND EXTRACT - THYROID					✓
ANTIOXIDANT	✓				
ANXIETY				✓	
BODY BUILDING				✓	
CIRCULATION				✓	✓
COGNITION	✓	✓	✓	✓	
DEPRESSION	✓	✓	✓	✓	✓
DIGESTION	✓			✓	
DIGESTIVE ENZYME SUPPORT				✓	
ENDURANCE	✓				
ENERGY	✓	✓	✓	✓	
ERECTILE DISFUNCTION				✓	
FAT BURNING	✓			✓	
FERTILITY	✓	✓	✓		
FLUID RETENTION	✓				
GLUTATHIONE SUPPORT	✓				
HOT FLASHES	✓	✓	✓		
IMMUNITY	✓				
INFLAMMATION				✓	
INSULIN SUPPORT				✓	
JOINT SUPPORT	✓				
LACTIC ACID FLUSHING	✓				
LIBIDO	✓	✓	✓	✓	
LIVER DETOX	✓				
LOWERS BLOOD SUGAR				✓	
MENOPAUSE	✓	✓	✓		✓
MENSTRUAL BLOOD FLOW					✓
MEMORY	✓	✓	✓	✓	
METABOLISM					
MOOD SWINGS	✓	✓	✓	✓	
MOTIVATION		✓	✓		
MUSCLE AND BONE MASS		✓	✓	✓	
NATURAL ESTROGEN THERAPY		✓	✓		
PMS	✓	✓	✓	✓	
REDUCES CORTISOL LEVELS				✓	
STRESS	✓	✓	✓	✓	
TESTOSTERONE SUPPORT FOR MEN		✓	✓	✓	
VAGINAL DRYNESS	✓	✓	✓	✓	
CONTAINS DHEA		✓	✓	✓	
CONTAINS PREGNENOLONE		✓	✓		
NO ESSENTIAL OILS		✓			

VITALITY™ USAGE GUIDE

	CALMING/SLEEP	CLARITY (MENTAL)	ENERGY	METABOLISM	WOMEN HORMONES	MOBILITY (MUSCLES/JOINTS)	BRAIN HEALTH	CIRCULATORY	DIGESTION (ENZYMES/GUT)	ENDOCRINE	IMMUNITY	LYMPHATIC	LIVER	RENAL/URINARY	BLADDER	KIDNEY	NERVOUS	RESPIRATORY	HAIR, SKIN, NAILS
BASIL VITALITY™		✓				✓					✓								
BERGAMOT VITALITY™	✓				✓					✓	✓								
BLACK PEPPER VITALITY™			✓	✓		✓			✓	✓	✓								
CARDAMOM VITALITY™		✓					✓		✓				✓				✓	✓	
CARROT SEED VITALITY™									✓				✓	✓					✓
CELERY SEED VITALITY™						✓			✓				✓	✓					
CINNAMON BARK VITALITY™			✓	✓				✓	✓	✓	✓								
CITRUS FRESH VITALITY™	✓		✓	✓					✓	✓	✓		✓						
CLOVE VITALITY™						✓		✓	✓	✓	✓			✓	✓				✓
COPAIBA VITALITY™	✓					✓				✓	✓			✓	✓	✓		✓	✓
CORIANDER VITALITY™	✓								✓				✓						✓
DIGIZE VITALITY™			✓						✓		✓								
DILL VITALITY™	✓							✓	✓				✓						
ENDOFLEX VITALITY™					✓					✓									
FENNEL VITALITY™			✓	✓				✓	✓	✓			✓						
FRANKINCENSE VITALITY™	✓	✓				✓	✓				✓						✓	✓	✓
GLF VITALITY™									✓		✓								
GERMAN CHAMOMILE VITALITY™	✓								✓				✓						✓
GINGER VITALITY™			✓			✓			✓	✓								✓	
GRAPEFRUIT VITALITY™	✓	✓	✓	✓						✓	✓	✓	✓	✓	✓	✓			
JADE LEMON VITALITY™		✓	✓						✓		✓	✓	✓	✓	✓	✓			✓
JUVA CLEANSE VITALITY™									✓		✓								
JUVAFLEX VITALITY™									✓		✓								
LAURUS NOBILIS VITALITY™					✓				✓									✓	
LAVENDER VITALITY™	✓	✓			✓	✓	✓	✓		✓	✓		✓				✓	✓	✓
LEMON VITALITY™		✓	✓					✓	✓	✓	✓	✓	✓	✓	✓				✓
LEMONGRASS VITALITY™		✓	✓			✓	✓	✓	✓	✓	✓	✓	✓	✓			✓	✓	
LIME VITALITY™	✓			✓					✓	✓	✓	✓	✓	✓				✓	
LONGEVITY VITALITY™							✓				✓								
MARJORAM VITALITY™	✓					✓		✓	✓										
MOUNTAIN SAVORY VITALITY™			✓			✓				✓	✓			✓	✓				
NUTMEG VITALITY™		✓	✓		✓	✓		✓	✓	✓	✓	✓	✓						
ORANGE VITALITY™	✓		✓					✓	✓		✓		✓	✓	✓	✓	✓		✓
OREGANO VITALITY™			✓			✓		✓	✓	✓	✓		✓	✓				✓	
PEPPERMINT VITALITY™		✓	✓	✓		✓	✓	✓	✓	✓	✓	✓					✓	✓	✓
ROSEMARY VITALITY™		✓	✓			✓		✓	✓	✓	✓	✓	✓	✓	✓		✓	✓	
SAGE VITALITY™		✓	✓	✓	✓				✓	✓	✓								
SCLARESSENCE VITALITY™					✓					✓									
SPEARMINT VITALITY™		✓	✓			✓		✓	✓	✓	✓								
TANGERINE VITALITY™	✓		✓					✓	✓	✓	✓		✓	✓	✓	✓	✓		
TARRAGON VITALITY™	✓							✓	✓	✓			✓						
THIEVES® VITALITY™			✓	✓		✓		✓	✓	✓	✓		✓	✓				✓	
THYME VITALITY™		✓						✓	✓	✓	✓		✓	✓			✓		

These statements have not been evaluated by the Food and Drug Administration. Young Living® products are not intended to diagnose, treat, cure, or prevent any disease. Please consult your medical doctor before starting any natural hormone therapy.

SUPPLEMENTS USAGE GUIDE

	FOUNDATION	CLEANSING	TARGETED	KID SAFE	MEN SPECIFIC	SLEEP	WEIGHT SUPPORT	ENERGY	HORMONES	MOBILITY (MUSCLES/JOINTS)	MILD LAXATIVE	BRAIN HEALTH	CIRCULATORY	DIGESTION (ENZYMES/GUT)	IMMUNITY	RENAL/URINARY/LIVER	RESPIRATORY	HAIR, SKIN, NAILS	BONES
AGILEASE™										√				√				√	
ALKALIME®										√		√		√				√	
ALLERZYME™														√					
AMINOWISE™										√									
BALANCE COMPLETE™	√						√							√					√
BLM™										√									
CARDIOGIZE™					√		√	√		√		√	√				√		
COMFORTONE®		√									√			√					
CORTISTOP®									√										
DETOXZYME®														√					
DIGEST & CLEANSE™		√												√	√	√			
ENDOGIZE™					√				√					√					
ESSENTIALZYME™														√					
ESSENTIALZYMES-4™														√					
FEMIGEN™							√		√										
ICP™		√									√			√					
IMMUPRO™						√									√				
INNER DEFENSE™	√														√		√		
JUVAPOWER®		√												√		√			
JUVATONE®		√												√		√			
K & B™														√		√			
KIDSCENTS MIGHTYPRO™	√			√										√	√		√		
KIDSCENTS MIGHTYVITES™	√			√															
KIDSCENTS MIGHTYZYME™	√			√										√					
LIFE 9™	√													√	√		√		
LONGEVITY SOFTGELS™	√											√	√	√					
MASTER FORMULA™	√							√		√		√	√					√	
MEGACAL™										√									√
MINDWISE™								√		√		√	√						
MINERAL ESSENCE™	√																√	√	√
MULTIGREENS™		√										√		√					
NINGXIA NITRO®								√				√	√						
NINGXIA RED®			√					√				√	√	√	√	√	√	√	
NINGXIA ZYNG™								√				√	√						
OMEGAGIZE3™	√											√	√					√	√
PD 80/20™									√							√			
PARAFREE™		√													√		√		
POWERGIZE™					√									√			√		
PROSTATE HEALTH™					√				√										
PURE PROTEIN™ COMPLETE			√				√							√					
REHEMOGEN™		√										√							
SLEEPESSENCE™						√	√									√			
SLIQUE® SHAKE							√							√					
SLIQUE® BARS							√												
SLIQUE® CITRISLIM							√												
SLIQUE® GUM							√												
SLIQUE® ESSENCE ESSENTIAL OIL							√												
SULFURZYME® (CAPSULES & POWDER)												√						√	
SUPER B™	√							√											
SUPER C™ (CHEWABLE)	√			√												√	√		
SUPER C™ (TABLET)	√															√	√		
SUPER CAL™ PLUS							√			√			√					√	√
THYROMIN™							√		√										

These statements have not been evaluated by the Food and Drug Administration. Young Living® products are not intended to diagnose, treat, cure, or prevent any disease. Please consult your medical doctor before starting any natural hormone therapy.

ADDITIONAL RESOURCES

୬

Get the Apps THE EO BAR AND LIVE WELL WITH YOUNG LIVING
Available for Apple and Android

ONLINE RESOURCES
www.facebook.com/JenOSullivanAuthor
www.facebook.com/groups/TheHumanBody
www.SparkDroppers.com (team site)
www.JensTips.com (YouTube)
www.JenOSullivan.com
@JenAuthor on Instagram
Podcast: Jen O'Sullivan Podcast
www.31oils.com

BOOKS AVAILABLE BY JEN
For bulk purchasing of any of her books please go to www.31oils.com

VITALITY: THE YOUNG LIVING LIFESTYLE
All about the Young Living lifestyle and products.
Available on Amazon and at www.31oils.com/vitality

THE RECIPE BOOK WITH JEN O'SULLIVAN
Over 250 recipes for essential oil enthusiasts. Recipes that work!
Available on Amazon and at www.31oils.com/recipe

THE ESSENTIAL OIL TRUTH: THE FACTS WITHOUT THE HYPE
48 micro lessons to help you understand the world of oils.
Available on Amazon and at www.31oils.com/truth

FRENCH AROMATHERAPY: ESSENTIAL OIL RECIPES & USAGE GUIDE
The essential oil users guide to proper use and dosage using the French
method of Aromatherapy with over 300 recipes.
Available on Amazon and at www.31oils.com/french

ESSENTIAL OIL MAKE & TAKES:
Over 70 DIY Projects and Recipes for the Perfect Class
Available on Amazon and at www.31oils.com/make-takes

LIVE WELL
FOR WELLNESS, PURPOSE, AND ABUNDANCE
PSK mini is Available on Amazon and at www.31oils.com/live-well

ESSENTIALLY DRIVEN
YOUNG LIVING ESSENTIAL OILS BUSINESS HANDBOOK
The quick guide to starting your business the right way.
Available on Amazon and at www.31oils.com/essentially-driven

66093625R00111

Made in the USA
Columbia, SC
16 July 2019